THIN and THINNER

Solutions to Permanent Weight Loss in
the Real World for Moms to Models…

If We Can Do It, So Can You!

By Ida Fiorella and Emily Fiorella

The authors of *Thin and Thinner* recommend that you discuss any ideas that you intend to use from this program with your physician prior to implementing the plan. We expressly disclaim responsibility for any adverse consequences following the commencement of the eating plans and lifestyle changes outlined in this book.

TABLE OF CONTENTS

www.thinandthinner.net

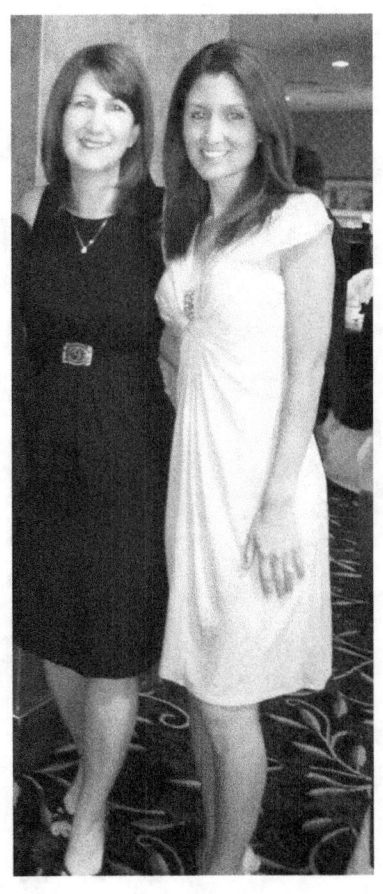

Discovering

the Fountain

of

THIN

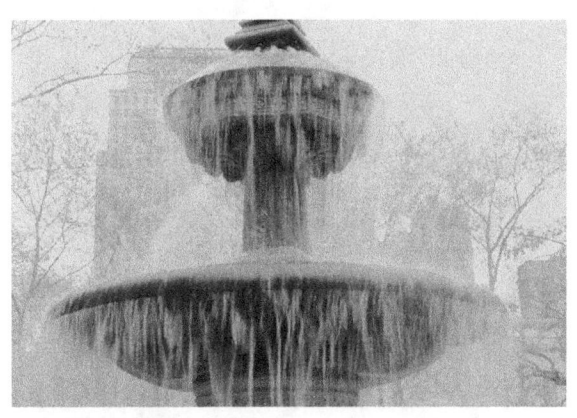

CHAPTER 1: INTRODUCTION

Who are we and why are we qualified to write this book? We are two regular people, mother and daughter. We are not scientists, nor are we doctors. We have battled the bulge since childhood, Emily (Thinner) for about 18 of her 28 years and Ida (Thin) for about 43 of her 56 years. Until now, neither of us had ever experienced a plateau where we stayed the same weight for any length of time. Both of us were either gaining pounds or losing them. We have read scores of diet books and have tried many over the course of time. We don't need to go for testing to find out if either of us has "the fat gene", all we need to do is to open our family photo album! Going by that—we're doomed! Our relatives, particularly those who have already "stuck their spoon in the wall", fall (or fell) into 2 basic categories: those that are on a diet and those that need to be. So, think of us as "experienced dieters" with 61 collective years of valid experience. We have successfully kept the weight off and have each maintained the same clothing size for 10 years. How have we done it? That is the subject of this book.

We have searched the web for many years, trying to find a longitudinal study of people who follow a low-carb diet. To date, we have not found one. Most studies end within a matter of months. Due to this lack of research, it is difficult to gauge the success of the program. No diet's effectiveness can be determined in the short term. Losing weight is a challenge. But, keeping it off is the true test of a diet's value. So, we have begun to study ourselves and represent a microcosm of an informal longitudinal study.

You likely know many people who have lost a significant amount of weight. But, have they kept it off? Probably, very few have. You, or they, may have even tried an approach similar to the one we are supporting here, but were not able to sustain it. It is our contention that it is not terribly difficult to lose weight. Going low-fat, low-calorie, running, and low-carb will all get you to your goal weight. However, the challenge is in keeping it off. Any diet that is not a life plan is truly not worth the effort.

One of us has reached her goal weight three times before discovering the approach to permanent and successful weight loss: twice on *Weight Watchers* and once on *The Bruce Lowell Fat Percent Finder* diet. In fact, Ida is a life time member of *Weight Watchers*. Notice the words "reached her goal weight" were not associated with the word success. Reaching the goal was not the success. If the weight had been kept off, that would constitute success. Slowly, but surely, each of these times, the weight would creep back up. The difference between this book and the hundreds of other books that are out there is that this one was written by 2 people who are genetically destined to be corpulent, given our western diet, who have successfully and happily kept the weight off for 10 plus years and are willing to share the experience. This book will equip you with all you realistically need to lose your excess weight and never gain it back. It provides the dietary and lifestyle changes for you to discover, realize, and sustain your ideal weight.

So, this is a diet book in that it explains what the ideal diet is for us and could be for you. But, it is not a diet book, in the sense of a temporary eating plan that ends when the goal weight is achieved. Anyone who thinks that once he/she reaches goal weight, the problem is solved is quite frankly—not the sharpest pencil in the box; but, will sooner than later be the fattest pencil in the box.

CHAPTER 2: THE SCIENCE BEHIND THE DIET

Here is the simplest explanation of the how the diet works. When carbohydrates are consumed, the body converts the carbohydrates into sugar (glucose). When glucose is present in the blood, insulin is released. The primary role of insulin is to take the sugar out of the blood. Some of the sugar is used for energy. The remainder is stored as fat. This is the same fat that we see on our abdomen, legs, and other parts of our bodies. It is also the fat that leads to heart disease. When it comes to simple carbohydrates, the truth is that our bodies are equal-opportunity fat storers. It does not matter whether the person is ingesting white bread, pasta, potatoes, or a 3 Musketeers Bar; the fat <u>will</u> be stored.

According to Gary Taubes, an acclaimed science writer and author of <u>Good Calories, Bad Calories</u> and <u>Why We Get Fat and What to Do About It</u>, "When insulin levels go up, we store fat. When they (insulin levels) go down, we mobilize it (fat) and use it for fuel." In the absence of carbohydrates, the body will utilize proteins and fats to produce energy. Consumption of protein and fat will not spike insulin levels the way that carbohydrates do. If insulin is not spiked, the body will not store as fat the calories consumed.

The whole premise is that you don't want to wake the sleeping giant, A.K.A. – insulin. To avoid doing so, you simply avoid sugars and starchy carbs. And, this is why the diet is sustainable for life. You do not need calorie counters, point systems, scales, or special pre-packaged foods. All you need to do is limit the carbohydrates.

This is the basic information that led us to embark upon a low-carb lifestyle. And, it has sustained us for the past 10 years and counting.

We would highly recommend that you look further into the science supporting the low carbohydrate lifestyle, for yourself. It will strengthen your resolve, as well as provide you with intelligent responses to questions by skeptics. The following recent books fully explain the science underlying the low carb plan:

Why We Get Fat and What to Do About It by Gary Taubes

Good Calories, Bad Calories by Gary Taubes

New Atkins for a New You by Dr. Eric Westman, Dr. Stephen D. Phinney, and Dr. Jeff S. Volek

Also, there are other excellent books, listed in the reference section of this book, which give further elaboration on the science behind low carb diets.

CHAPTER 3: HOW WE CAME UP WITH THE NAME OF OUR BOOK:

Thin and Thinner

For the past ten years, we, Ida (Thin) and Emily (Thinner), have followed the *Thin and Thinner* dietary and lifestyle plan. However, we have individually customized the program in order to accommodate our unique weight goals and lifestyles, and to sustain a lifelong commitment to low-carb living. Thinner's ideal weight and lifestyle require a more disciplined plan. Thinner eats 6 mini meals per day, has smaller portions that do not add unnecessary calories, and is diligent when it comes to exercise, trying her best to make it to the gym four or five times per week. These habits have allowed her to develop and maintain an extremely lean and healthy physique.

On the other hand, Thin's goals do not require such a stringent program. Thin eats three meals per day with at least the minimum amount of recommended protein, enjoys a glass of wine with dinner most evenings, and engages in a low key workout on an exercise bike several nights a week (or when she can); all the while, keeping an admirably thin figure and a level of health that has been charted in the top 5 percentile of the US population.

By following our plan, *Thin and Thinner,* you will soon be thin, and you will have the option to be even thinner if you choose to eat smaller portions and increase your level of physical activity. Both plans are outlined in the pages to follow.

CHAPTER 4: GOING AGAINST THE GRAIN

Before you get started, you have to ask yourself if this is something you are definitely ready for. At the moment, the low-carb lifestyle is somewhat out of the mainstream—"going against the grain". Low-carb living requires a true commitment. Alternating this plan with a low-fat program or any other diet, where starchy carbs and sugar are included, is a recipe for disaster. Low-carb living is a monogamous relationship. So, you need to decide if you are willing to give up breads, desserts, and potatoes in order to be thin, energetic, and healthy. If your answer is yes, then you are ready to read on because the first step to losing weight and keeping it off is having the right mindset. You will need to make a commitment to follow this plan as strictly as possible. We will help you along the way, as you read the pages to follow. We encourage you to learn from our normal, every-day life experiences and utilize our meal plans, recipes, menu ideas, grocery lists, and charts which will help you to personalize the plan to your own lifestyle. Once you learn the program, it will become second nature, and you won't need to write anything down.

But, at the outset, a word of caution is needed. Don't let others bring you down. We have both had experiences where people aggressively tried to persuade us to abandon the low-carb diet. Perhaps they felt that we were a threat to their grains and pasta. Or maybe they were trying to save us from what they perceived as an unhealthy plan. Thinner has been ridiculed for being thin and has lost a friend or two due to envy and jealousy. But, thankfully, she never lost her resolve or her faith in the program. Our best advice is to surround yourself with supportive people who build you up. They will be very impressed as they see you not only take the extra pounds off, but keep them off.

If You'd Like to be
Thin...

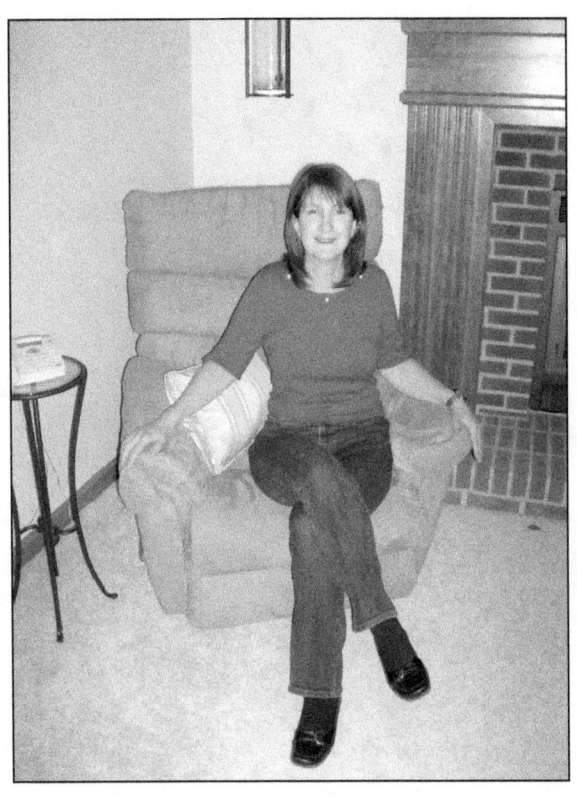

CHAPTER 5: THIN'S JOURNEY TO MAINTAIN A HEALTHY WEIGHT

Since I can remember, I have always fought the battle of the bulge. Being a very young girl, I became aware that I was chubbier than most of the other children around me. By the age of 13, I began to buy those little Dell books near the cash registers in grocery stores that suggested diet plans for losing weight. I remember diets such as the egg and orange diet—Ugghhh!

In my teen years, I was slender, but not skinny. I watched what I ate and walked or biked everywhere, maintaining a healthy 117 pounds. My husband and I married early, and we had our first child when I was age 20. After the pregnancy, I was unable to get my weight under 132 pounds. If I did not watch everything that went into my mouth, I would gain weight. If I was not actively dieting, my weight would continue to creep up. I never experienced a plateau. This had and has continued to be my reality. If I did not regularly diet, I am quite certain that I would be morbidly obese. I was annoyed, but resigned to the inevitable.

Then, 2 ½ years later in 1978, we had our second child, and my new post-pregnancy weight was 167! According to the recommended height/weight charts, I either needed to gain 8 inches in height, or lose 35 pounds. Since the first was not possible, I knew I needed professional help. I joined Weight Watchers. Within 6 months I went from 167 pounds to 117. I kept the weight off for one full week. Then, I continued very gradually to gain it back. Thus began a cycle of yo-yo dieting that continued until 2001.

I lost the pounds once more on Weight Watchers and once again on a low fat/low calorie diet (1350 calories and 43 grams of fat). Each time, I reached my target, but very gradually gained it all back, plus more. After these diets, my weight spiked into the 160s.

In the years 1998 and again in 2000, I was the mother of the bride, and I was very motivated to lose weight for those bridal pictures. At that time, whole wheat and fiber were touted as the answer. I switched from white bread and white rice to whole wheat and brown rice, and I began to eat a variety of beans. I followed the suggested meal plans and portion sizes in the books. But, to my dismay, the best I could do was 155 pounds for the first wedding and 151 pounds for the second.

By early 2001, I reached a turning point in my life, determined to find the answer for permanent weight loss. I decided that I needed to find something that I could realistically do for the rest of my life. The diet had to be a way of life, not something temporary that would end when I reached my goal weight. While on vacation in Florida, I found a book that revolutionized my thinking about diets. The book is titled, <u>Life without Bread: How a Low-Carbohydrate</u>

Diet Can Save Your Life, by Christian B. Allan and Wolfgang Lutz. The basic principle of the book is that a low-carbohydrate/high-protein diet can improve the quality of your life and help you to maintain a healthy weight.

After reading this book, I purchased other books that followed this premise. First, I read Dr. Atkins' New Diet Revolution by Robert C. Atkins. I followed this text with The Protein Power Life plan by Michael and Mary Eades. The Schwarzbein Principle by Diana Schwarzbein and Lick the Sugar Habit by Nancy Appleton also found their way onto my bookshelf. Each of these was significant in giving me the foundation, tools, and resolve necessary to completely overhaul my diet for life. A bibliography at the end of this book lists these as well as a plethora of other great books we have read which offer deep scientific explanations regarding metabolism, diet plans, suggested exercise routines, recipes, and more.

Each book gave excellent advice, but I needed to modify each to fit into my life. My meals became a very interesting and enjoyable experiment. The weight was finally sliding off. When certain foods caused my weight loss to stall, I did not view the situation as a failure, but as a learning experience. I knew that I was in this for the long haul, and I was already doing maintenance while losing the weight!

Within 6 months, my weight dropped from 167 pounds (and rising) to 129 pounds. My clothing size dropped from a size 14 to a size 6. I had to bring all of my 8s, 10s, 12s, and 14s that were in the closet to the Good Will truck. It was so much fun to go shopping and have choices. Usually, I would try on 20 items until I found something that looked decent. Now, everything looked good. I had to choose which articles of clothing looked the best. Now, at age 56, I am still a size 6. I haven't outgrown one item in the closet. The initial new wardrobe cost a bit, but I am saving a bundle by maintaining the same size. There is also a lot more room in the closet!

CHAPTER 6: HOW THE DIET HAS CHANGED THIN'S LIFE

Besides helping me to maintain a healthy, normal body weight and consistent clothing size (from size 14 to size 6), eating a low-carbohydrate diet has positively impacted my life in the following ways:

- dramatic increase in energy level
- significant reduction in food cravings
- fewer incidents of brain fog
- vastly improved cholesterol level without medication
- better health

Nothing in life happens in isolation, and any diet will have consequences far beyond just weight issues.

<u>Dramatic Increase in Energy Level</u>

Before I understood the importance of controlling carbs, I had significant problems with energy. I knew I had less pep than others. As a young adult in my 20s, I'd go shopping with my mother who was 30 years older than me. I had great difficulty keeping up with her. I was constantly telling her that she walked too fast.

At around three o'clock every day, I was completely exhausted, feeling the force of gravity weighting me down. I thought I needed to eat something to energize myself. I'd grab whatever was easily available. Often, I would eat a half of a bag of potato chips thinking it would give me enough energy to cook dinner. But, somehow, it never worked. I forced myself to do what I needed to do and suffered in silence.

Then, I became an elementary school teacher in a public school. I got through each day on shear adrenaline. But, then, 3 o'clock would roll around. The students were gone, and I would be sitting at my desk, staring at the chalkboard, wondering how I was going to get up to erase it. Work that should have taken an hour at most, would take me three hours to do. The custodians always commented that I was so dedicated, leaving at 6:00 p.m. every night. They had no idea that I was just trying to stay afloat.

Exercising was completely out of the question. I could barely keep the house clean, leave alone start an aerobic workout! If it were not for my husband, we would have had to hire a cleaning lady. I could never have managed the house on my own. I knew that exercising would actually energize me, but I was too sapped to start. It was truly a vicious cycle.

But, once I started limiting my carbohydrates, my energy level was transformed. Truly, the most important benefit to me, even greater than the weight loss, was the improvement in my stamina. In 2001, I remember laughing as I ran around the house cleaning and organizing everything. I went out and bought an exercise bike, which I plopped in front of the television set in my bedroom. I had so much energy, I didn't know how to get it out of my system! I haven't experienced that drag-down feeling in 10 years, and my life is remarkably better. I can walk for miles without tiring,   I run up and down the stairs easily, not letting items heap at the base of the steps in order to save trips, and I am always looking for ways to stay active, whether it's at the gym, taking hikes, going for long walks, or golfing at the local par 3. I have cut at least 2 hours off of my time spent at school, just in getting my after school work done in a reasonable amount of time. Now, my energy level is as good, if not better, than any of my friends and family.

Significant Reduction in Food Cravings

For as long as I can remember, I was the queen of carbohydrates. I had a huge sweet tooth. I loved candy, doughnuts, chocolate cake—especially frosting, and all kinds of sugary treats. I would even crave sweets as my main course. Sweet and sour chicken was my favorite dish. I also loved fresh bread, pizza, ravioli, lasagna, and pancakes. I could go on and on.   I had great difficulty limiting my portions. Once I started eating, it was very difficult to stop. As a teacher, students would often give me a box of chocolates as a gift. I remember coming home and eating 7 or 8 pieces in a row. Then, my face would start to perspire, and I would need to lie down.

Now, I only eat an occasional sugar-free sweet. I have no desire to eat any of the items above. If I am with a group that is enjoying a treat, I have a low carb treat, or I have a bite of theirs. It is amazing how one bite is completely satisfying. It gives the same wonderful taste without the calories or cravings.

I make sure that everything I eat tastes good. Yet, I never have a problem stopping when I am full. My body tells me when I have had enough. That is a major advantage of being on a low carb diet. The carbohydrate addiction is not an issue.

Elimination of Brain Fog

One of the most annoying problems that I have experienced in my life is what many have termed "brain fog". This term refers to the inability to process information. Prior to my low carb diet, there seemed to be no rhyme or reason to when this would happen. I would be trying to listen to someone, but I could not follow the full line of thought. At those times, my responses would be limited to very simple answers with little or no elaboration.   Sequences would be hard to comprehend.

As I have become better at following the low carb plan, my instances of brain fog have diminished. I recently asked my doctor about this, and he gave the following explanation. A university study, focusing on the blood flow to the brain, was done, where a subject was given a tablespoon of sugar. The blood flow to the man's brain was reduced by 38 % shortly after he ingested the sugar. A normal person's blood pressure will pump the blood back up to the person's brain. But, my doctor has theorized that since I have quite low blood pressure, my body does not pump the blood back up to the brain as quickly.

I have been likely depriving my brain of its vital blood supply. He has since advised me to never eat simple carbs—ever!

Improved Cholesterol Level

Several years ago, my doctor sent me for routine cholesterol screening. The results came back, indicating that I had elevated cholesterol and was borderline for needing cholesterol-lowering medication. I opted not to take the medication. Since then, I began my low-carb life.   All testing done after I started limiting my carb consumption has shown dramatic improvement. I went for check-ups a few years ago. Both my family practice physician and my gynecologist sent me for blood work. Both affirmed that my cholesterol levels are wonderful. According to my physicians, my cholesterol HDL and LDL are perfect. In fact, one doctor told me that my cholesterol is so good that the only way that people like me die is if they get run over by a bus.

Better Health

Having been on a higher protein/low-carb diet for 8 years, I was a little uneasy about being tested two years ago for a life insurance policy. I have heard so much about the impact of protein on the kidneys, and I wondered if there has been a toll on any of my organs. This was the moment of truth. You will understand how vastly relieved I was when the 4 page fine print analysis of my testing came back with glowing results. An EKG, blood samples (testing

19 different levels), and urine testing (which examined 9 different levels), as well as height, weight, and blood pressure screening all attested to my excellent health. I was given elite status and a reduced rate for life insurance. My financial planner said his office cheered when the results came in because it is so rare to get such a good rating. I am in the top 5% for good health!

Another result on my diagnostic sheets was my BMI (body mass index). My BMI is listed as 22.6. 8 years ago, my BMI was 28.5. To put this in perspective, a healthy BMI ranges from 18.5 to 24.9. A BMI of 25 is considered overweight, and a BMI of 30 defines obesity. I was certainly overweight, and nearly obese. The health risks associated with obesity could be the topic for another book.

CHAPTER 7: THE DIET IN A NUTSHELL

- 3 main meals a day

- approximately 21 g (usually about 3 ounces) of protein per meal

- non-starchy green vegetables (about 1 cup per day, many unlimited)

- healthy fats

- 2 snacks per day

- no more than 12 net carbs* at any one meal

- no more than 25 net carbs per day (excluding non-starchy green vegetables)

- main meals spaced 4 to 5 hours apart

- never go more than 6 hours without eating

Breakfast	21 g protein	healthy fats	up to 12 g carbs with daily limit – 25g
Lunch	21 g protein	healthy fats	up to 12 g carbs with daily limit - 25 g
Snack	up to 7 g protein	healthy fats	up to 12 g carbs with daily limit – 25 g
Dinner	21 g protein	healthy fats	up to 12 g carbs with daily limit – 25 g
Snack	up to 7 g protein	healthy fats	up to 12 g carbs with daily limit – 25 g

* Net carbs = total carbs – fiber
Note: Each ounce of meat or cheese is equivalent to about 7 grams of protein.

CHAPTER 8: THE PLAN

What to Eat:

PROTEIN: 3 – 5 ounces per meal (9-11 ounces
recommended per day)   [7 grams = 1 oz.]

- beef
- fish
- shellfish
- poultry
- pork (including ham and bacon)
- lamb
- veal
- other meats
- eggs (substitute 1 egg for 1 ounce of protein)
- cheese and cream cheese
  (limit cottage cheese and ricotta cheese)
- protein powder (approx. 21 grams of
  protein per serving)
- peanut butter or almond butter
  (substitute 2 tbsp. for 1 ounce of protein)

FAT: (Use as much as needed, but don't go crazy!)

- olive oil
- canola oil
- butter (regular)
- any other healthy oil (no transfats)
- mayonnaise
- salad dressing (with 2 carbs or less per serving)

NON-STARCHY VEGETABLES: (eat about 1 cup per day—unless *)

- artichoke hearts
- asparagus
- broccoli
- brussel sprouts
- cauliflower
- celery*
- cucumbers*
- eggplant
- lettuce*
- mushrooms*
- onions (all kinds)
- peppers*

- spinach
- squash (spaghetti squash, summer squash, and zucchini)
- string beans
- tomatoes
- water chestnuts
- any other green vegetable

*unlimited

SNACKS: 2 of the following per day:

---

1. Fruits: (1/4 cup of berries)
   - strawberries (5 large or 10 medium)
   - blueberries
   - raspberries
   - blackberries
2. Nuts and Seeds: (1/4 cup)
   - almonds
   - macadamia nuts
   - peanuts
   - pecans
   - pistachios
   - sunflower seeds
   - walnuts
3. Sugar Free Treats:
   - candy (1 or 2 pieces)
   - ice cream (1/2 cup)

- Jell-O (1 serving)
- pudding (1 serving)

4. low-carb protein bar with 12 net carbs or less per serving (2 times per week)

5. any no sugar added product with 12 net carbs or less per serving (1 time per week)

6. flax chips or other snacks with 4 or fewer carbs

DAIRY:

- half and half or cream (amount needed to lighten coffee)
- sour cream (1/4 cup occasionally)
- whipped cream (on berries)
- yogurt (plain or sugar free—3 carbs or less per serving, once per day)

OTHER ITEMS:

- ground flaxseeds or Anutra
- spices
- unsweetened cocoa powder

BEVERAGES:

- coffee
- tea
- water

- unsweetened iced tea
- sugar free drinks

ALCOHOL: (Be careful. Alcohol will slow down your
metabolism.)

- dry wine, red or white
  (4 oz.–up to once per day)
- any non-sweet liquor
  (1 oz.–up to once per day)

SOY:

- Shirataki tofu noodles (thin noodles packed in water, taste just like angel hair pasta)
- soy milk (1 cup)

PREFERRED SWEETENERS:

- Stevia
- Truvia

PREFERRED THICKENING AGENTS

- Guar Gum
- Xanthan Gum
- Thick N' Thin—Not Starch
- (avoid thickening with corn starch or flour)

Other Notes:

Since this is a permanent lifestyle diet, everything that goes in your mouth should taste good.
This may require enhancing foods with, for example, a bit of low sugar barbecue sauce or gravy onto
meat. An occasional tablespoon of such items will
not throw you off.

Foods to Avoid

Avoid all carbohydrates that are not on "The
Plan". Do not eat...

potatoes
rice
pasta
beans (legumes)
bread or baked goods
bagels, pastries, or muffins
starchy vegetables such as corn and peas
sugar in any form
honey
molasses
syrup
candy
desserts of all kinds
flour
breaded or battered food
oats
other grains
cream-based soups

sauces and gravies thickened with flour or corn starch

milk (fat free, low fat, and whole)

fat-free cheese

low fat and fat free salad dressings

fruit yogurt

fruit (other than berries)

dried fruit

juice

any sugar-sweetened beverage

cashews

pumpkin seeds

popcorn, chips, and crackers

Also, limit diet soda since it leads to carbohydrate cravings.

CHAPTER 9: THIN'S TYPICAL MEAL CHOICES

Breakfast Ideas

protein shake
yo'tmeal
ham and egg cup
vegetable or cheese omelets
bacon, ham, or sausage and eggs

Lunch Ideas

chicken salad
egg salad
hamburger/no bun
salad topped with chicken, shrimp, or beef
open chicken souvlaki
chicken wings
broth-based soup with added chicken
omelets
left-overs from previous dinner

Dinner Ideas

3 – 5 oz. Meat or fish	1 Cup of Vegetables	2 Cups of Salad
• filet mignon • meat sauce with tofu noodles • beef veg. soup • barbecued chicken • roast chicken with cheese sauce • chicken soup • almond-crusted chicken tenders • barbecued ribs • pork tenderloin • pan-seared shrimp • almond-crusted tilapia	• roasted green beans • asparagus w/ Hollandaise Sauce • Asian style spinach • mashed cauliflower • sautéed broccoli with garlic and olive oil • zucchini patties • spinach bars • roasted broccoli	• romaine lettuce • tomatoes • onions • green olives • shredded cheese • sliced almonds • Good Seasons Mild Italian Salad Dressing

Sample Menu 1 (Thin)

Breakfast	10 g net carbs

yo'tmeal (recipe in this book)
2 small cups of coffee with half and
half

Lunch	0 g net carbs*

Chicken salad made with 1 small
chicken breast mixed with 2 tbsp. of mayonnaise
and ¼ cup of chopped celery

Snack:	4 g net carbs

¼ cup of almonds
2 small cups of coffee with half and half

Dinner	6 g net carbs*

3 - 5 oz. of filet mignon (recipe in book)
1 serving of zucchini patties (recipe in book)
1 cup of romaine lettuce with tomatoes, onions,
   and shredded cheddar cheese
2 tbsp. Good Seasons Mild Italian Salad Dressing
4 oz. dry white wine

Snack:	4 g net carbs

1 cup of herbal tea
1 square of home-made
   sugar-free chocolate
   candy (recipe in book)

Total for day: 24 g net carbs*

*This carb count does not include the non-starchy green vegetables. This menu includes about 6 additional net carbs from the non-starchy green vegetables.

Sample Menu 2 (Thin)

| Breakfast | 10 g net carbs |

yo'tmeal (recipe in this book)
2 small cups of coffee with half
and half

| Lunch | 0 g net carbs* |

Open chicken souvlaki (no pita)

| Snack: | 4 g net carbs |

1 ounce of hard cheese
2 small cups of coffee with half
and half

| Dinner | 11 g net carbs* |

8 jumbo pan seared shrimp
(recipe in book)
1 cup of roasted green beans
(recipe in book)
4 oz. dry white wine

| Snack: | 2 g net carbs |

1 cup of herbal tea
1 chocolate crunch cookie
(recipe in book)

| Total for day: 25 g net carbs* |

*This carb count does not include the non-starchy green vegetables.
This menu includes about 10 additional net carbs from the non-
starchy green vegetables.

Sample Menu 3 (Thin)

| Breakfast | 2 g net carbs |

3 eggs and 2 slices of bacon
2 small cups of coffee with half and half

| Lunch | 0 g net carbs* |

cheeseburger (no bun) with lettuce,
onion, and tomato slice
side salad with blue cheese dressing

| Snack: | 2 g net carbs |

3 mini cheese pizzas (recipe in book)
2 small cups of coffee with half and half

| Dinner | 10 g net carbs* |

roast chicken breast with cheese sauce (recipe in book)
1 cup of sautéed broccoli (recipe in book)
10 medium strawberries with whipped cream

| Snack: | 11 g net carbs |

1 cup of herbal tea
½ cup of low carb ice cream

| Total for day: 25 g net carbs* |

*This carb count does not include the non-starchy green vegetables. This menu includes about 9 additional net carbs from the non-starchy green vegetables.

CHAPTER 10: THIN'S GUIDE TO PORTION CONTROL

- Never eat till you are stuffed. Listen to your body. It will tell you when you are comfortably full.

- Don't let yourself get so hungry that you are out of control. Feel free to snack whenever you are hungry.

- Don't worry about consuming butter and approved oil. Use as much as is needed to make your food taste great. But, don't overdo it. Fat is loaded with calories. You will have extra energy, but you will need to burn it off.

- Try to keep to the lower end of the serving spectrum on days when you will be a slug.

- Conversely, you may eat on the higher end of the serving spectrum on days when you will be getting plenty of exercise.

- Pay attention to feelings of hunger and satisfaction. It's a good idea to take breaks while eating. If you are no longer hungry, stop eating.

- A protein serving ranges from 3 to 5 ounces. 3 ounces is about the size of a deck of cards. 1 ounce of meat, fish, or cheese is about

7 grams. So, eat at least 21 grams for each of the 3 meals.

- As a general guideline, eat approximately one cup of non-starchy vegetables per day. Salad greens are basically unlimited.

- If you are going to overeat—do it on green (or non-starchy) vegetables. Roast them, steam them, or eat them raw.

- Limit snacks to 2 servings per day.

- Total carbs may vary, depending on your individual metabolism and your activity level.   Try not to exceed 25 carbs per day.

CHAPTER 11: THIN'S ANSWER TO "WHAT IF I AM HUNGRY IN BETWEEN MEALS?"

The rule of thumb is to schedule meals every 4 to 6 hours. If I am eating an adequate amount of protein and fat at meals, the thought of eating again usually doesn't occur to me until just before the next meal.   But the problem with this strategy is that in the real world, we can't always eat within this time frame. Because we do not live in a perfect world, snacks become necessary.

I eat breakfast at 6:45 a.m., consisting of yogurt/flax cereal (yo'tmeal recipe in back of book) and coffee. My scheduled lunch is at 11:00 a.m. I am just ready for a meal by then, so I have no need for a snack between breakfast and lunch. But, between lunch and dinner, it is a totally different story. From 11:00 lunch, there is usually a 7 hour gap before dinner. We typically eat around 6:00 p.m. Between 3:15 and 5:00, I am usually ready to eat something.

Below are the snacks that I eat which carry me till dinner. But, a note of caution is needed. I am often tempted to eat more than 1 serving. If I do not give into temptation, I am usually just fine. But, when I do indulge in a second serving, then I am not hungry for dinner. There would be no problem if

I skipped dinner. But, who ever skips dinner? Not me, and it's a "no brainer" as to where those extra calories are going to land—somewhere in the vicinity of my hips and thighs. So, the moral of the story is—just eat one serving of snack in between each 2 meals. The objective of eating the snack is to hold us over until the next meal.

After dinner, I usually do not eat much because I am not hungry. If I am with friends, I will sip a glass of dry wine and nibble on some nuts or cheese. But, I usually indulge myself with a chocolate square or chocolate crunch cookie in the evening. Both recipes can be found in this book. I make a batch which will last more than a month.

Except for green non-starchy vegetables, the net carbs in each item below need to be counted towards the daily 25 g net carb limit. Those snacks with no mention of carbs do not contain carbohydrates. I usually have coffee or tea with my afternoon snack which will add 1 g of carb for each cup.

Suggested Snack Servings

- 1 ounce of hard cheese (about 1 slice or seven ½ inch cubes)

- ¼ cup of nuts (pistachios, almonds, pecans, peanuts, walnuts, or macadamia) or sunflower seeds. These nuts average about 2 g net carbs per serving. The sunflower seeds are 3 g net carbs per serving.

- 2 tablespoons of almond butter or peanut butter (4 net carbs* per serving)

- 2 mini pizza snacks (recipe in back)

- 1 hardboiled egg

- celery and dip (I only eat dip that contains 4 g net carbs or less per serving.)

- Starbucks tall Frappaccino light (occasionally). It has 16 g net carbs. But, this particular beverage doesn't derail the program if consumed 2 or 3 times per month.

- chocolate squares (sugar-free fudge) (recipe in back) (4 g net carbs)

- 1 or 2 chocolate crunch cookies (recipe in back) (2 g net carbs per cookie)

- ½ of a low carb protein bar (See bar for carb count.)

- homemade cheese crackers* (recipe in back)

- sugar-free pudding with 1 scoop of protein powder** (See carton for carb count.)

- sugar-free Jell-O with whipped cream (See carton for carb count.)
- ½ cup of low carb no-sugar added ice cream (once or twice a week at most) (11 g net carbs for Edy's No Sugar Added Vanilla)
- ¼ cup of blueberries (4 g net carbs)
- 5 large or 10 medium strawberries with whipped cream (6 g net carbs)
- 1 or 2 pieces of sugar free candy (occasionally). I would save this treat until nearly bedtime since it may spike carb cravings to some extent. (See package for carb count, and see note below regarding sugar alcohols.)
- flax chips or other snack with 4 or fewer net carbs

* When calculating the carb content, the important number is the net carbs. This is found by subtracting the grams of fiber from the grams of carbohydrates. For example, a peanut butter jar states that each serving contains 6 total grams of carbs and 2 grams of dietary fiber. $6 - 2 = 4$. So, that peanut butter has 4 net carbs per serving.

** no more than 2 net carbs

Note: Sugar alcohols are rather controversial. Many low carbers subtract the sugar alcohol content from the total carb content in figuring the net carbs. I have trouble maintaining weight when I do so. Now, I just count the sugar alcohols as regular carbs, working them into my 25 carb daily limit. But be careful with them and use sugar alcohols sparingly. They can cause stomach discomfort.

CHAPTER 12: HOW THIN IS ABLE TO STAY ON THIS DIET FOREVER

This is the most important chapter in the book. Without an understanding of how to maintain the weight loss, the rest of the information is useless. What follows are the nuts and bolts of how to normalize your low-carb lifestyle in a carb crazy world.

If you live alone, cooking only for yourself and never eating out at restaurants or at the homes of others—no problemo! Skip this chapter and head for the recipes! Everyone else will do well to learn from our experiences.

When I began my low carb lifestyle, the most challenging part for me was the social aspect. This included

- vacations
- restaurants
- entertaining friends and family
- cooking for family
- being entertained at someone else's home
- baby and wedding showers and other parties
- food gifts
- unexpected events

I will share what has worked for me in helping these aspects to be non-issues.

Often on vacation, we stay at a hotel. In my pre-low-carb days, I would inevitably gain 5 pounds for every week away. Since starting my new life plan, the following strategies have helped me to either maintain or gain 1 or 2 pounds at most in a week.

- We avoid the elevator. Whenever we stay at a hotel, motel, or inn, we use the stairs whenever possible. The elevator is only used in high rise situations.

- I always plan ahead. We request a refrigerator and stop at a local grocery store on our way to the hotel. We stock the fridge with low carb yogurt, cheese, and spring water. I also bring protein powder, flax, and olive oil to make breakfast. If we feel like going out for breakfast, that is fine. But this way, I don't have to have eggs every morning. I also make sure that I have a few measured servings of nuts and a few protein bars on hand for any days where there is a large span between meals.

Eating at restaurants is easy. For breakfast, there are usually at least 5 omelets to choose from. Also, I could order bacon or sausage and eggs. For lunch, I might order an open chicken souvlaki, a bacon cheeseburger with no bun, chicken satay lettuce wraps, or a specialty salad with shrimp, chicken, or steak, just to name a few. At dinner, we usually forgo the bread basket. Dinner typically begins with a house or Caesar salad (no croutons). The main course consists of fresh seafood or meat with a green vegetable. Most restaurants will only offer a starch as a side. But, if you ask, they usually will bring you a delicious green vegetable instead. I usually have spinach, green beans, asparagus, or broccoli. Sometimes they offer something really interesting like a zucchini and cauliflower medley. I often have a glass of dry wine and end the meal with a cup of coffee. If my husband gets dessert, I get my standard "taste". It is one bite, but just as good as his whole serving. He gets 95 % of the calories, and we both have the same delicious taste in our mouths! It's a really good deal for me!

When entertaining company, I try to make everyone happy. I have a number of satisfying dishes that the low carb and non-low-carb crowd can eat. If we are having a cold cut platter, I might eat slices of provolone cheese wrapped around slices of roast beef, slathered with a little mayonnaise. If we are having pizza and wings, I'll rip the cheese and pepperoni off a slice and have that with 5 or 6 chicken wing drumsticks, dipped in blue cheese, of course! If it's a barbecue, I'll have the barbecued chicken and salad. I skip the corn on the cob and the baked beans. Often times, the meal is one that is just perfect for me, but for the company, I'll add in a potato dish, crackers with the cheese, and a scrumptious bakery dessert. But, Thanksgiving Day is unique. Every year, I have 25 to 30 guests for Thanksgiving dinner. For this particular meal, I make all of the traditional dishes. We usually will have smashed cauliflower or spinach pie as one of the vegetables. But, during the feast, I eat a little of whatever I feel like eating. It is once a year, and the holiday is an expression of thanks to God for the bountiful harvest. It is not a day to prohibit anything!

Dinners at our house had always been balanced. Prior to my low-carb days, the evening meal consisted of meat, a starch, and a frozen or canned vegetable. A good portion of the work went into preparing the potato, rice, or pasta side dish. Thus, there was little thought given to the vegetable. The vegetable was a duty, something to be tolerated, a necessary evil. The adults ate them to set a good example for the younger generation, and the children ate their age. For example, if you were 5, you had to consume 5 string beans. The older one got, the greater was the objection to this system.

Today, meals at our house still consist of 3 parts: meat, an interesting side salad, and a delicious vegetable dish. In fact, the vegetable is the most coveted of the platters on the table. Whether it's roasted zucchini, sautéed spinach, roasted green beans or asparagus, or fresh broccoli sautéed in oil and garlic, there are never leftovers. No one leaves the dinner table hungry, and everyone raves over our delicious, satisfying meals. Life is good at dinner time!

Also, I don't bake anymore. If a dessert is in our home, it is brought in by someone else, or it has been made at the local bakery. In past years, I baked often. My husband would eat a tiny piece of the cake or brownies, or a few cookies, and I would eat the rest. The accessibility and aroma from freshly baked treats would be too much of a temptation for me, and I know not to subject myself to it, and no one in my house expects me to.

When I am invited to someone else's house for dinner, dessert, or snacks, some preparation is necessary. First of all, **EVERYONE I KNOW MUST KNOW THAT I AM ON A LOW-CARB DIET.** Somehow, this fact manages to come up in the first few hours of my meeting someone. It should certainly come up before I am intimate enough to be invited over to someone's house. This prevents the host/hostess from being insulted or upset that I am refusing one of his/her special dishes. I have come to realize that I cannot eat high carb items that people make just so as not to hurt their feelings. But, more importantly, this provides my friend with the information needed to provide acceptable dishes for his/her guests. I would feel terrible if I invited someone to my home for a prime rib dinner, only to find out when she arrived that she is vegetarian!

My husband and I are blessed with a large family and many friends. We are often invited to their homes. All of them have always been and continue to be extremely considerate, and subsequently, I have plenty of great foods to enjoy. One of my friends even buys low-carb fudgesicles so that I can have dessert with them, and she'll make eggplant parm for me when they are having pasta. The only trouble is that everyone wants the eggplant parm! My other friends and family are just as considerate, offering shrimp platters, and a variety of acceptable foods. Another newer friend had invited our group for a spaghetti dinner. I mentioned to her a few days in advance that I was bringing a little baggie of cooked low-carb pasta if she could save out a little of the sauce. She was more than happy to comply. I was glad because her sauce was awesome!

When I am invited to someone's home, I always ask what I could bring. If the hostess happens to mention the menu and I then determine that there would be nothing there that I could eat, I make sure that I bring something that I could enjoy. I'll often show up with a veggie platter, nuts, or a cheese platter. Everybody loves it!

Bridal showers and baby showers are sometimes a bit of a challenge for me. Often times, the only beverage they have is that sweet punch. I am not a fan of tap water, so sometimes I can get really parched at these events. I am learning to bring a small bottle of spring water. Sometimes, horror of horrors, we are presented with a tea party. It starts out with scones accompanied by Devonshire cream, followed by dainty tea sandwiches, and ending with a tray of delectable desserts. There is not one morsel of food that I can consume. At these events, I visualize that I am Sam Adams, ready to organize a group of rebels to toss the entire contents of the tea party into the Boston Harbor! But, as I sit there fantasizing, I am fairly content, because I knew enough to have eaten a light meal before I left the house. I can at least enjoy the tea!

High-carb items are offered to me on a regular basis. As a school teacher in a building with nearly 700 students, I am given at least one cup cake every day. I would be as big as a house if I consumed these goodies. I keep a box of baggies in the classroom, just for these gifts. I bring them home to my husband who enjoys such treats now and then, since I don't bake anymore. Gift boxes of candy are accepted graciously. They are certainly useful to put on the table when company arrives.

Finally, life is filled with surprises. I have spent whole days in emergency rooms or hospital waiting rooms. I have been pleasantly surprised to find that nuts are often an option in the vending machines. A few years ago, my mother was in the hospital for nearly two months. I would go right from work each day and spend every weekend there. I packed a large snack when I knew that I would not likely have an opportunity to step out for a meal.

Whether the car breaks down, or the plane is delayed several hours leading to an extended airport stay, acceptable food is usually available. One night, my dinner consisted of a bag of peanuts from the airport convenience mart. It wasn't the ideal answer. But, it was the best I could do. A high carb meal would have drained me of energy, spiked my cravings for more food, induced brain fog, and messed up my metabolism for the next 2 to 3 weeks. All that considered, the nuts were just fine.

CHAPTER 13: THIN'S EXPERIENCE WITH EXERCISE

As an elementary school teacher, I work about 50 hours a week. Add to this a husband, 3 daughters, 6 grandchildren, live-in parents, sisters, nieces, nephews, and the dearest friends anyone could have. Needless to say, I don't have much time for exercising. I have tried gym memberships with really good intentions. I start out being consistent for about 2 months, and then I rarely ever go back. Life gets in the way.

But, the metabolic benefits of exercise, as well as the enhancement in mood and energy, make it vital to me. So, what has worked for me for the past 10 years is a small exercise bike with a back rest. I keep it in my bedroom near the television set and the phone. While I pedal, I catch up on all of my phone calls and television viewing. In fact, the only time I ever watch TV is when I am on the bike. I know that it is not the ideal cardio workout. But, it does get my heart rate up over 100 beats per minute, and it certainly is better than nothing—which is what my only alternative would be. My goal has been to pedal for about one half hour, 4 days per week. Some months out of the year, this works well. While there are intervals during certain hectic months that I rarely have time for any exercise at all.

I have learned that a 25 minute workout, combining the elliptical and treadmill, give me a far superior workout. A few years ago, I managed to join and go to the local gym about 4 times per week, and I really started to notice results on the scale. I lost a few pounds, my clothes were looser, I had even more energy, and I actually looked forward to my workouts. I kept this up for about 6 months. But, then, life became hectic at work, and my trips to the gym tapered off to nothing.

I still use the exercise bike about 4 times per week, and I have now added ten minutes of floor exercises. I am still thin, and I continue to wear a size 6, but I am not as toned as when I did the cardio workout at the gym.

I am hoping to make a deeper commitment to exercising. I need to set it as a priority. But, in the meantime with this inconsistent workout pattern in my life, I am very thankful that I have an eating plan that is effective. Maintaining a healthy weight is not dependent on my level of physical activity, and I am grateful that my exercise roller coaster has little impact on my size.

If You'd Like to be

Thinner...

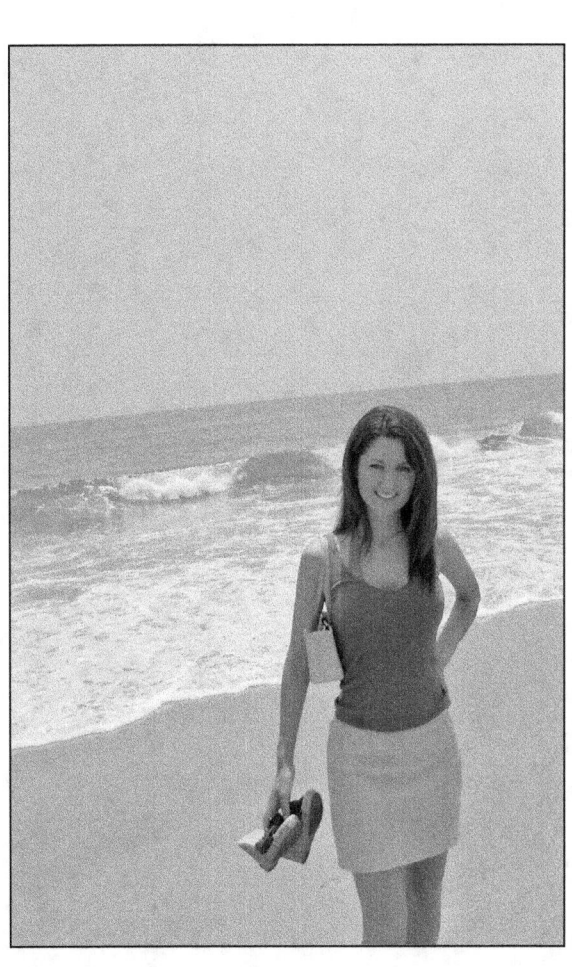

CHAPTER 14: THINNER'S STORY

I had been health conscious for as long as I can remember. But, I lost control when I went away to college and moved in with my friend's family. I no longer had access to the healthy foods my mother provided me with at home. My friend had a super high metabolism and could eat everything under the sun without gaining weight. I was surrounded with her mom's homemade cookies, brownies, cakes, pies, and cinnamon rolls, as well as doughnuts, cereal, pizza, potatoes, and pasta. But, I felt confident that I had strong will-power and could withstand the consequences of indulging by keeping my portions under control. Nevertheless, after only a few months of living with Betty Crocker, I had gained my "freshman 15"—every girl's worst nightmare.

I had been hearing that consuming large quantities of sweets and starches were unhealthy, and that eating an adequate portion of protein was important, but I did not understand why. I was constantly craving carbohydrates and always thinking about my next meal. I remember being incredulous that thoughts of food were seriously taking over my life.

For a time, I lost my motivation to lose weight altogether since controlling my portions was not working. I began to feel self-conscious while eating anything that was not considered healthy in front of others because everyone knew I was trying to shed a few pounds. Consequently, I started to hide what I ate. I would make sandwiches, pour bowls of cereal, grab a bag of cookies, and take the food to my room to eat so no one would see. I would overeat and feel a terrible sense of guilt. Sometimes, I would delude myself into thinking that it was okay because I could just take a laxative to reverse everything I just ate. The next day, I would feel sick and drained. And then I would have to eat even more for energy and drink a ton of fluids to rehydrate. It was a vicious cycle. I was exhausted and depressed.

My mom mailed me the Atkins book, and I tried to follow it. But, I kept going off the diet due to the non-accessibility of appropriate foods. I didn't have my own refrigerator and relied on meals prepared by my friend's family. Consuming the few items that were low-carb became tedious and boring after a while. And while going on and off the diet, I was mixing high amounts of carbs with large amounts of protein and fats. This led to me gaining even more weight.

The issue that slowly began to surpass the desire to be thin was my need for energy. I constantly felt lethargic and was plagued by brain fog. It was difficult for me to focus, and I was consumed with thoughts about my next meal, hoping that that would rectify the situation. I had heard that exercising helped to increase stamina. So, one day my friend and I started running together. I could not even make it to the end of her cul-de-sac. Our runs turned into walks, and then after about a month, I just gave up.

I also had major digestion problems, too. I was not regular, and that led me to start taking laxatives. Soon, I became reliant on them.

I regularly purchased fitness magazines and read diet books to learn all that I could to help me. But, nothing was effective for me.

I was self-conscious, insecure, and certainly not the same happy person that I had been before going away to college. I wanted so badly to be pretty, energetic, and successful. Being a fashion design major, I had a stylish wardrobe, but I kept to the basics because I did not have the confidence or the figure to pull off the trendier outfits.

I have a small frame and never thought that I could look fat, but I was what you would call a "skinny" fat person. I woke up one morning, looked in the mirror, and noticed that my face was chubby and sagging, I had elastic marks around my waist from my underwear being too tight, and my arms were flabby. I was finally determined to change. I wanted to look lean and healthy. I wanted to be hot! And, that's when I called home and started to work with my mom to make some major changes in my dining habits.

With my mom's support, I was able to figure out an eating plan that could work as a way of life. We were able to come up with foods and recipes that satisfied our cravings, but also were high in protein, fiber, healthy fats, as well as being low in carbs. Along with this, I stopped taking a specific type of birth control pill that was elevating my blood sugar level, I started taking a multi-vitamin with digestion support, and I slowly started a consistent exercise regimen.

Since then, I have taken off the excess weight that I gained in college and have the body that I always dreamed of. I am happy, energetic, and successful. When I get off track, it is short-lived, and I get right back on. Nowadays, I am always prepared for any social situation. I definitely do not consider myself on a diet; rather, I am just living a low-carb lifestyle. I love my life, I'm truly happy, and I hope to be an inspiration to others.

CHAPTER 15: THE DIET IN A NUTSHELL
(THINNER'S PLAN)

- Up to 6 mini meals a day

- Protein ranges from approximately 5 – 15 g per meal (consuming at least 50 g per day)

- Carbs can range from 0 - 15 g per meal, not to exceed 40 g per day (excluding non-starchy green vegetables)

- On days without exercise, carbs are restricted to no more than 25 g

- Sip on hot green tea, water, have coffee as a treat, occasionally drink no-sugar- added cranberry juice (diluted with water), and limit alcohol consumption to one night a week.

- Eat small portions, consistently throughout the day. Don't let yourself get too hungry and never eat until you're stuffed.

Mini meal #1 Breakfast	<15 g protein	healthy fats	0 to 15 g carbs per mini meal no more then 25 – 40 g per day
Mini meal #2 Mid-morning snack	<5 g protein	healthy fats	0 to 15 g carbs per mini meal no more then 25 – 40 g per day
Mini meal #3 Lunch	<15 g protein	healthy fats	0 to 15 g carbs per mini meal no more then 25 – 40 g per day
Mini meal #4 Mid-afternoon snack	<5 g protein	healthy fats	0 to 15 g carbs per mini meal no more then 25 – 40 g per day
Mini meal #5 Dinner	<15 g protein	healthy fats	0 to 15 g carbs per mini meal no more then 25 – 40 g per day
Mini meal #6 Late Night Dessert	<5 g protein	healthy fats	0 to 15 g carbs per mini meal no more then 25 – 40 g per day

For the details, see Chapter 8: *The Plan*.

CHAPTER 16: TYPICAL MENUS (THINNER)

Sample Menu 1 (Thinner on a Day without Exercise)

| Breakfast | 10 g net carbs |

Perfect Protein Shake (recipe in this book)
1 serving of Chai tea (recipe in this book)

| Mid Morning Snack | 2 g net carbs |

¼ cup of mixed nuts

| Lunch | 0 g net carb* |

2 egg, ham, and cheese omelet

| Mid Afternoon Snack | 6 g net carbs |

Sugar-free pudding cup mixed with ½ scoop of protein powder

| Dinner | 3 g net carbs |

Chicken Alfredo over tofu noodles (recipe in this book)

Late Night Dessert	4 g net carbs

Chocolate Square (recipe in this book)

Sample Menu 2 (Thinner on a Day with Exercise)

Breakfast		9 g net carbs

Yo' tmeal (without oil, recipe in this book)
1 serving of Chai tea (recipe in this book)

Mid Morning Snack		7 g net carbs

Flax crackers topped with 1 tbsp. almond butter

Lunch		0 g net carb*

¼ cup seasoned ground beef

Mid Afternoon Snack		6 g net carbs

Peanut Butter Melt (recipe in this book)

Dinner		4 g net carbs

Teriyaki Skirt Steak

Late Night Dessert		6 g net carbs

Sugar-free vanilla ice cream topped with cinnamon

Sample Menu 3 (Thinner on a Day with Exercise)

| Breakfast | | 10 g net carbs |

Sausage Egg and Cheese Breakfast Sandwich
(recipe in this book)
1 Chai tea (recipe in this book)

| Mid Morning Snack | | 6 g net carbs |

Cannoli Snack Mix (recipe in this book)

| Lunch | | 16 g net carbs |

Starbucks Tall Coffee Frappaccino
Light + protein

| Mid Afternoon Snack | | 0 g net carb* |

String cheese

| Dinner | | 0 g net carb* |

Dining out: Ahi Tuna with veggies or Filet
with veggies

| Late Night Dessert | | 6 g net carbs |

½ cup strawberries with whipped cream

CHAPTER 17: EXERCISE–THINNER USED TO GET TIRED JUST THINKING ABOUT IT

When I was a little girl, I could outrun everyone. When I was in kindergarten, I was often the last kid standing in freeze tag and always the first to finish when racing to the stop sign. But as time went on, I lost my speedy momentum. I remember in ninth grade gym class being tested for speed in running a mile. I ran the first lap around the track and walked the last three. Come to think of it, I think I skipped my last lap, and the gym teacher let it slide because all the other kids had finished. By that time, I had lost any inclination to join competitive sports. So, I got a job instead…at a bakery.

I now realize that my eating habits, which incorporated cereal for breakfast, Ramen noodles for lunch, cereal for a snack when I got home from school, and then pasta for dinner almost every night, seriously impacted my energy level. I was eating almost no protein (which is necessary for the body to function properly), no vegetables except for the occasional salad, and rarely any nuts or fruit.

Now that I get adequate amounts of protein, vegetables, healthy fats, nuts and berries, my stamina has increased. I currently enjoy running 2 to 4 miles or spending 20 minutes on an elliptical four to five times a week. I don't need long strenuous workouts. I can usually work up a sweat and burn a ton of fat calories in twenty minutes.

But, it's important to know that I don't <u>need</u> to work out to be slim. At times in my life when I am unable to work out, I'm just a little more strict about my carb intake, and I stay about the same size.

However, without exercise, I don't feel the same. I truly enjoy the mental benefits that come along with cardiovascular exercise. It's a natural anti-depressant, and scientists say it increases brain function and memory, as well. With exercise, I sleep better and longer, and I credit my workouts for elevating my self confidence. It's also a time for reflection and prayer. Since experiencing these benefits, I've become passionate about getting them. It's a natural high, an exhilaration that I hope everyone will experience within their lifetime. So, it should not come as a surprise that during those times when I am unable to exercise, I am very anxious to get "back on the exercise wagon".

Although exercise hasn't been necessary for either of us to lose weight on our diet, I would encourage everyone to become physically active for the following reasons:

- You only have to work out for half the time as your counterparts to get the same effect. Because you don't have as many carbs to burn, your body goes directly into fat burning mode. Most people need 20 minutes of rigorous exercise to burn through their carb stores, before they begin melting fat.

- Exercise can significantly improve your cardiovascular health, as well as your energy level and productivity. We can both attest to this!

- Exercise allows you to moderately increase your carbohydrate consumption without gaining weight. When I am regularly exercising, I can enjoy an occasional higher carb treat because it will be burned off quickly.

- Muscle increases your resting metabolism. Your body's metabolism stays revved for hours after a workout, keeping you in fat-burning mode (This should make you want to jump out of your seat and start exercising right now!)

- The more weight you lose from low-carb dieting, the more inclined you'll be to exercise, and the more consistent you are with exercise, the easier it will be to make it a part of your everyday life.

Here's the bottom line: a combination of a low-carb lifestyle and a twenty minute exercise routine will turn you into a fat burning machine. It's helped me to lose weight fast and more importantly to keep it off.

CHAPTER 18: THINNER'S ADVICE ON HOW TO SATISFY YOUR SWEET TOOTH WITHOUT GOING OFF THE DIET

As the low-carb diet evolved, so did the popularity of sugar-free snacks. The benefit that sugar-free snacks have to low-carb dieters is that they are made with sugar alcohols or artificial sweeteners which have a minimal impact on blood sugar/insulin. The artificially sweet indulgences have less effective net carbohydrates per serving, and they are lower on the glycemic index. The glycemic index refers to the impact of food on blood sugar.

You can find almost all of your favorite sweet products in a sugar free version. Everything from a variety of sugar-free cookies, assorted chocolates, sugar-free maple syrup, sugar-free ice cream, sugar-free JELLO, sugar-free pudding cups, sugar-free jam, and even sugar-free gum drops!

But, you have probably heard the old cliché', "If it's too good to be true, it probably is." This seems to be the case with sugar alcohols. When consuming more than one serving of a product containing sugar alcohols, the most commonly used varieties all have similar side effects such as gas, bloating, laxative effect, and diarrhea. The artificial sweeteners actually trick our bodies into thinking we are ingesting real sugar, stimulating the release of insulin, which can cause cravings for more carbohydrates.

Another type of sweetener to be weary of can be found in the majority of your favorite junk foods as well as popular "health" foods (Go figure!). It's high fructose corn syrup, which is used by most manufacturers because it is the least expensive of all sweeteners. The danger of HFCS is that it stimulates the production of a hormone that increases hunger and appetite. So, it makes you feel hungry even when you're not! Some experts in the field of nutrition cite high fructose corn syrup as a leading cause of obesity. There is also evidence that it is linked to diabetes. Initially, it received a healthy rap because it is naturally found in fruits and honey. But, it is not so healthy after it has been processed. Please pay attention to food and beverage labels to avoid consuming this at all costs.

The only sweetener I use that has none of the side effects above is Stevia, and it's unfortunate that there aren't many treats on the grocer's shelves sweetened with this. It is all natural. It comes from the *Stevia rebaudiana* plant, and it is 30 times sweeter than sugar, so you only need to use a tiny bit. Stevia has zero calories, it doesn't adversely affect blood glucose levels, and it may actually lower your blood glucose levels. It even has been found to significantly reduce the development of plaque to help combat cavities.

You can find Stevia in health food stores or even in the health/whole food section of your local grocery store. You'll notice in our recipe section that we prefer to use Stevia and Truvia (which contains Stevia) as our preferred sweeteners.

CHAPTER 19: THINNER'S THOUGHTS ON CONSTIPATION AND ELIMINATION

Constipation is one of the most uncomfortable conditions I have experienced. With constipation, I have felt weighted down, my stomach protruded out, and the number on the scale started creeping up.

Pre low-carb diet, I had gone through a very long period in my life, where I wasn't regular. I was having a bowel movement only once or twice a week. I knew I had to do something about it. I tried increasing my water intake, drinking prune juice, taking magnesium supplements, chewing on fiber tablets, and mixing fiber powders into my beverages and cereal, none which worked. Then, I turned to laxatives, and that did the job. Wow, I felt great! The weighed down feeling disappeared along with my waistline, and I loved it. So, I continued to use laxatives, pretty much to the point where I was dependent on them.

I did this for a little over a year, but I knew deep down that this was not healthy. I started researching the consequences of relying on laxatives. These include abdominal cramping, muscle spasms, irregular heartbeat associated with an insufficient amount of electrolytes, chronic pain and other problems associated with the health of one's colon.

As I was transitioning to my new low-carb lifestyle, I slowly weaned myself off the laxatives. I began to notice that my elimination problems were subsiding due to my elevated metabolism and consumption of higher fiber foods such as vegetables, berries, and nuts. Since incorporating the following into my daily routine, my days of constipation are firmly in the past.

- ☐ Daily multi vitamin with ECGC extract
- ☐ Sipping on hot green tea
- ☐ Using Stevia as a sweetener (aids in digestion)
- ☐ Having Yo' tmeal for breakfast or Detox Smoothie (see recipe's)
- ☐ Consuming olive oil (acts as a lube)
- ☐ Eating plenty of dark green vegetables
- ☐ Exercising (walking, running or elliptical) at least 4 times per week
- ☐ Using an occasional stool softener when needed (doesn't cause dependency)

Now my system is working just fine. Every morning, the first thing I do when I wake up is take my multi with ECGC extract, and I know that I'll be marching straight to the lav within minutes.

I need to mention that Thin has stayed regular using only the yo'tmeal, olive oil, and green vegetables. She has not needed to try anything else.

I believe that it is important for each of us to recognize and do something about constipation if we have it. Remaining constipated can cause blood sugar levels to severely fluctuate and lead to more problems. Add to this the fact that anything that remains in the colon will get reabsorbed into the body. As a rule of thumb, it is considered healthy to have anywhere from 3-12 bowel movements per week.

Living Low-Carb

in

the Real World

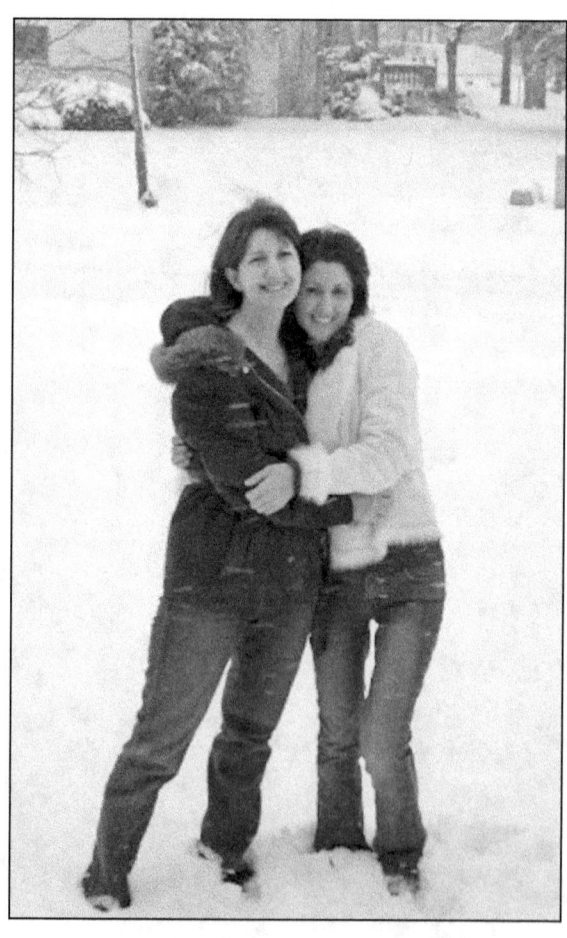

CHAPTER 20: BEVERAGES

Thin and Thinner have somewhat different prac-tices with regard to drinking. As with the other chapters in this book, we share this information to give a full account of what has helped us to thrive on a low carb diet for life.

<u>Water</u>

Both of us believe that staying hydrated is impor-tant. But, neither of us is conscious of a particular amount that we consume per day. We do try to pay attention to when we are thirsty and readily have spring water or purified water on hand to enjoy. Thin drinks at least 48 ounces per day, and Thinner drinks at least 2 glasses per day. One of Thinner's glasses of water has 2 ounces of unsweetened cran-berry juice, added for variety.

<u>Alcohol</u>

The most important fact to know about alcohol is that it puts "fat burning" mode on pause until the alcohol is used up. Dry wine is the preferred source, followed by unsweetened liquor, then light beer. Thin has a glass of dry white wine about 5 times per week. Thinner drinks twice a week. She prefers a couple of glasses of dry wine or vodka on the rocks with unsweetened soda water.

Coffee

Coffee on any diet has always been a controversial issue. Some argue that it negatively affects blood sugar levels/insulin, and some say it improves it. If you've been drinking coffee forever, we don't believe that you need to give it up, just don't overdo it. Thinner feels that it's a contributing factor to belly fat and prefers hot tea over coffee. But, she does have an occasional cup. Thin enjoys about 4 cups a day. To lighten the coffee, we use half and half. It adds 1 carb per cup to our daily carb count. But, cream would be even better. It has zero carbs. We rarely put milk in coffee since it has more carbs. Thin enjoys coffee without sweetener. It took her a few weeks to get used to it. Thinner recommends Stevia extract.

Tea

Thin and Thinner enjoy herbal teas, as well as regular tea. Thinner drinks 4 cups of hot tea each day, while Thin has an occasional cup. Both sweeten the tea with liquid Stevia. Thinner, occasionally, tops her tea with whipped cream. Both drink unsweetened iced tea with liquid Stevia (about 5 drops).

Other Beverages

Thinner enjoys an occasional cup of diet cocoa or sugar-free soy milk. She also will stop for a Starbucks Coffee Frappaccino light (grande) with a scoop of protein powder as a filling lunch about one time per month. Thin has an occasional cup of diet cocoa in the winter months and enjoys a tall Starbucks Coffee Frappaccino light a few times per month.

CHAPTER 21: VARIETY IS THE SPICE OF LIFE

One of the most common reasons people are unable to adhere to the low-carb lifestyle is the lack in variety of food choices. If you're only going to find 3 or 4 meals that you enjoy on this diet and recycle them day in and day out, chances are you're not going to enjoy them for very long. Also, you will be missing the nutrients that you can only get from eating a wide variety of foods. Soon, your body will start feeling deprived of these nutrients, and food cravings will arise.

To be successful on this diet for the rest of your life, you don't have to become a chef, but you are going to have to learn your way around the kitchen. If you can chop vegetables, measure portions of fruits and nuts, boil water, and operate a blender, you already possess the skills needed to make just about all of our recipes! Thinner has lived on her own for several years, and these are the skills that have gotten her through.

Next you have to be sure your refrigerator and pantry are stocked with low-carb friendly foods so that you can avoid the "there's nothing to eat" excuse. Refer to our grocery list, and make it a routine to visit the grocery store every week to buy fresh meats, veggies, fruits, and dairy. You will find that your shopping trip is primarily along the perimeter of the store. Rarely will you be needing to visit the inner aisles.

Also, Thinner picks a day, every other week, to go to her favorite health food store. She enjoys going to the health food store because she somehow always discovers some new low-carb treat that she had never tried before, adding even more excitement and variety to the program!

It's best to find at least 3 to 4 different meals that you like for breakfast, several lunch options, and even more dinner ideas. If you are having problems imagining different types of foods that you'll look forward to eating, look at our meal planning section. Here are some of Thinner's favorites:

Breakfast:
- yo'tmeal*
- sausage egg n cheese on a low-carb muffin*
- protein shake*
- low-carb French toast* & side of sausage

Lunch:
- low-carb macaroni n cheese with chicken*
- bacon and zucchini stir fry*
- everything salad*
- chunky chicken, vegetable soup*

Dinner:
- Ahi Tuna Sashimi
- Asian Teriyaki Skirt Steak*

- Chicken Pizzaiola*
- Peanut butter, coconut, chili, lime Chicken*

Dessert:
- Sugar free ice cream sundae
- Chocolate Squares*
- Berry-protein smoothie*
- Sugar free chocolate peanut butter frosting

* Recipes in book

One very helpful strategy is to freeze leftovers in individual freezer containers for future lunches and dinners. Also, we have at times made a month's worth of meals on a Sunday afternoon. We freeze them in individual containers and microwave them for lunches and dinners. We have found these strategies to be extremely helpful in adding variety, particularly to lunch options.

CHAPTER 22: GOING OUT TO EAT

Dining out can be challenging and quite tasteless on most other diets. If counting calories and fats is the objective, it is nearly impossible to stay "legal". You can't see calories, nor can you taste them. And, for the most part, you can't see fats. Most dieting diners are subjected to a plate of dry, tasteless broiled meat, a baked potato without butter (What's the point?), and a salad with fat-free dressing (Note: All fat-free dressings should be outlawed!). Who could possibly enjoy such a meal? We wonder how long a person could sustain such a plan.

On the other hand, low carb dieters enjoy delicious meals created by chefs at local restaurants. Making selections is not difficult. You would not be able to see or taste the calories or fats, but you can sure see and taste carbohydrates! That's a large part of what make low carb diets so effective as a lifestyle. Because there is little difficulty in identifying them, carbs are easier to avoid. You wouldn't need to put on your reading glasses to see the pieces of rice, potatoes, or noodles floating in a bowl of soup, nor would you need supersensitive taste buds to determine that the raspberry vinaigrette is loaded with sugar. You might ask if the chicken is breaded, or if the soup is cream based. But, that is usually the extent of the questions. You do not need to ask the server if you could have a list of all the ingredients that went into your meal, the specific quantity–how many cups, tablespoons, or ounces of each ingredient, as well as the number of calories and fat grams per serving! It would be virtually impossible to follow such a diet plan for the rest of your life if you ever wanted to eat out again. We do not want to give the impression that eating out is "a free-for-all" on a low carb diet. But, in comparison to other diets, low-carb living offers significant advantages.

In avoiding carbs at restaurants, there are a few obstacles to circumvent. Below are the strategies that work for us. Follow these simple dining-out tips and join us in staying Thin or Thinner forever.

Low-Carb Friendly Options/Recommendations for Dining Out

Appetizers

It is fairly easy to determine whether or not an appetizer is low carb because, typically, they are described in great detail on restaurant menus. Also, the portion sizes are usually pretty small, or meant for sharing, so you can't do too much damage in the appetizer department. Here are some apps we order most.

- Calamari (ask to prepare without the breading)
- Chicken or Beef Skewers

- Chicken Wings
- Salsa or Guacamole (Ask for cucumbers or celery to dip)
- Shrimp
- Cheese and Fruit plate
- Stuffed peppers (stuffed with meat or cheese-not breading)
- Mozzarella and Tomato (caprese salad)
- Tuna Sashimi
- Sushi Rolls (Even though they are rolled in rice, these do not seem to spike our insulin!)
- Chicken Satay

Soups / Salads

Generally, the thicker the soup, the more it's loaded with carbs. Most cream-based soups are thickened with flour or starch which are ingredients that add loads of carbs by the spoonful. So, when ordering, we ask the waiter if the soup is cream-based, and if it is, we avoid it.   We stick to broth-based soups. Some of our favorite soups are French Onion (without the bread), Japanese clear soup, and vegetable beef or vegetable chicken (without noodles). A thinner lobster bisque is also a hit with us.

Salads are delicious, interesting, and safe to order, as long as we forgo the croutons, oriental noodles, craisins, and mandarin oranges that are nestled in some of the more exotic ones.   We also avoid low-fat dressings which usually contain large amounts of sugar to compensate for the lack of fat content. And, of course, we avoid the sweet dressings. Topping our "Most Unwanted" are sweet-and-sour varieties, raspberry vinaigrette, honey-mustard, and French dressing.   We've found that many dinner salads can contain as much as 20 – 50 grams of hidden carbs. We don't need them.   Those carbs are definitely overkill on a masterpiece. We enjoy creative salads topped with toasted almonds, pecans, pine nuts, hearts of palm, artichoke hearts, avocado, water chestnuts, olives, bacon, blueberries, and shredded cheeses. We play it safe with dressings such as oil and vinegar, Italian, ranch, non-fruity vinaigrettes, and blue cheese.

Main Course

We opt for any protein entrée' such as steak, seafood, chicken, eggs, or tofu. The main courses to avoid are pasta-based dishes, anything that's breaded, and anything drenched in a sugary syrup or sauce such as sweet and sour chicken. If we can't avoid getting anything without the breading, we can usually scrape it off. Often times, we will order items served over pasta or rice. We simply ask the server if they can substitute spinach or broccoli for the carbs. They are usually happy to comply. Interesting sandwiches can often be served without the roll. At Italian restaurants, Thin sometimes orders roast chicken breast, and asks for a side of tomato sauce. She cuts up the chicken and pours on the sauce. It is a delicious alternative to spaghetti! When it comes to sides, we avoid the starches: rice, bread, pasta, and potatoes. If they won't substitute, we request that they just leave those items off the plate. But, most restaurants these days will substitute extra veggies for the side.

Dessert

Dessert could be the most tempting of all courses. If we're at a restaurant with someone who orders the most decadent of desserts, such as the mile high pie or chocolate lava cake, we limit ourselves to a bite and reward ourselves with a low carb treat when we get home.   (We find that it is very important to keep the house stocked with acceptable goodies.)   Some restaurants offer berries with whipped cream. This is a perfectly fine dessert for us! When we choose this dessert, our dining mates usually look longingly at our dish, wishing they had what we are having!

If at an ice cream parlor, many now cater to the low-carb/diabetic population with sugar free options. Try ordering sugar free ice cream with sugar free hot fudge, peanut butter topping, or whipped cream. (This can be ordered at many ice cream parlors such as Friendly's, Cold Stone Creamery, and Kiliwins).

When you're on the go and craving something sweet and cold, try a Starbucks blended coffee frappaccino light. The plain coffee flavor has the least amount of carbs of all the fraps. Plus, you can now add protein powder to your frap in most locations for a mini meal replacement.

In Summary

We eat out often. Yet, as we have learned to follow these guidelines, dining out has not hindered us in maintaining our low-carb lifestyle or our weight. In fact, it is truly the only weight loss plan that we know of that is truly restaurant-friendly. When going out to eat, we do not alter our eating plan, nor do we sacrifice on taste. Any diet plan that would not work in a restaurant setting, or one that would force us to eat tasteless foods, would be impossible to sustain for life. We are constantly thankful that we have found an eating plan that works in any situation.

CHAPTER 23: TIPS TO STAY MOTIVATED AND CONTINUE LOW-CARBING FOR LIFE

Have confidence in the lifestyle. Understand that a low-carb diet will work. Leave no room for doubt. When you have the complete confidence in the effectiveness of any tool, you are more likely to continue using it. Just because you hit an occasional plateau, it does not mean that the diet plan is not working. Eating low-carb will absolutely lead to successful weight loss. But, the time frame is different for everyone, and knowing that you are on the road to thinness will prevent you from giving up.

Make it your hobby. Read as much as you can about this lifestyle in books and on websites. Enjoy it! Experiment with recipes, keep diaries, and reflect on what's working and what isn't from a scientific/ inquisitive perspective. As you gain knowledge, you will refine your eating habits. Early on in Thin's low carb life, she had the idea that onion rings would be an excellent substitute for a baked potato when dining out. And during this time frame, she could not understand why she had reached a stubborn plateau in her weight loss. It was only when she happened to look it up that she discovered the carb count on a serving of onion rings—55 carbs! Needless to say, Thin stayed clear of onion rings after that, and opted instead for extra veggies!

When you have a setback, see it as a learning experience. Setbacks are useful in strengthening your resolve. Thin's team at work had the practice of bringing in a delicious cake to celebrate each time it was someone's birthday. Although Thin was following a low carb plan, she would rationalize that this was a special day and she could have a slice. Within minutes of consuming a modest piece of cake, Thin would experience brain fog and a sick feeling of sluggishness. Her energy level was soon depleted, she could not carry on intelligent conversations with others, and it would ruin the rest of her birthday. To make matters worse, it would take a few weeks to see any weight loss on the scale. It seemed as though no matter how diligent she was in avoiding carbs, the insulin, released due to that cake, was busily storing everything in her body as fat. After a few years, she realized that the cake was not worth the consequences on her birthday. Now, her team orders out for lunch on birthdays, instead of getting cakes. Thin enjoys a delicious order of extra crispy chicken wings with celery and blue cheese! And, in the evening, her birthday dessert is a low carb cake or strawberries with whipped cream.

Your desire to lose weight and your willingness to do so has to come from within. The low-carb lifestyle depends upon a lifelong commitment, with no turning back. It requires a quality decision, steadfast resolve, and the realization that this is the only way for you to achieve permanent weight loss. It will necessitate effort; but, the outcome and lifelong benefits will far outweigh any efforts involved.

Set realistic short term and long term goals. Studies have shown that the main characteristic that separates high achievers from low achievers is the presence of clear, specific goals. Write down your goals and steps to achieving them. Visualize the outcome. Here are some goal setting ideas:

- Create an image of what you want to look like and why. Imagine specific situations where your new look might benefit you—perhaps on the job, while being part of the dating scene, or to improve certain aspects of your relationship with your significant other.

- Define a time frame that allows for the activities that will help you to achieve your desired results. This includes grocery shopping, preparing meals, exercising, charting your progress, and researching new recipes. One of the great saboteurs of any diet is lack of time. If allowances are not made for the tasks needed to maintain a lifestyle, it is bound to fail. We have heard many times from those who have been unsuccessful in losing weight that they simply did not have time to prepare special foods, and that they only had time for quick meals and convenience foods. What goes into the body plays such a huge role in the quality of life, and it is amazing to us that so many would not prioritize this with their time.

- Form a plan of how you're going to reach your goal. Learn your approved foods and those that are restricted. Develop a personalized meal plan, use the grocery lists in the back of this book, and decide how you are going to incorporate exercise. Eventually, you won't have to keep a written plan. It will become second nature, and it is only then that the diet truly morphs into a lifestyle.

- Invent strategies and solutions to overcome obstacles you might come across, such as sharing the lunch room at work with a group of anti-low-carbers. You might start bringing in healthy alternatives to share, such as interesting cheeses and nuts, fresh veggies, home-made low carb chocolates, berries with whipped topping, or you may decide to simply limit the time you spend there. Another obstacle could be that you might be hungry at 3:00 p.m. at work each day and need to figure out what snack to pack, so that you won't be tempted to eat the first food that comes along.

- Realize how achieving your specific goal will help you feel and act, versus just how it will make you look. You will have increased energy, confidence, and stamina leading to greater effectiveness and efficiency in life.

Thin and Thinner have experienced great benefits to health and brain function, along with many other advantages.

It's not what you eat that will contribute to your weight loss; it's what you don't eat. Have you ever heard someone say, "I'm following this new diet, and I had a salad with grilled chicken for lunch today and salmon with veggies for dinner. But, I don't understand why I'm not losing weight." Well, what else did that person eat that day? A carb-filled muffin for breakfast and cookies for dessert? We are a bit cynical when someone says the low-carb diet doesn't work for him. Well, did he really do it? If we hired a private investigator, would we find out that the complainer ate a candy bar because he was stressed or that there was nothing else to eat at the continental breakfast so he had a bagel with cream cheese? These slips are not tolerable on a low-carb diet. Tendencies such as this, which stray from the plan, will make anyone gain weight, unless he or she is involved in strenuous daily exercise.

While in the losing-weight phase of this low-carb lifestyle, going "off the plan" during one meal has set Thin back 2 or 3 weeks. So, we understand that faithfulness to the program is essential. One event of carb-overload could ruin several weeks' worth of progress.

Make sure to have a substitute for your favorite indulgences. This way you won't ever feel deprived.

The guide which follows may assist you while overcoming cravings. Thinner calls this a comfort food converter. See her examples below:

Craving	Substitute
French Toast	You can make this at home with lower-carb bread or if you're at a restaurant, order it to be made with whole wheat bread, along with sugar free syrup, and a side of protein such as sausage or eggs—any style.
Pasta	Tofu noodles (found in health food section of grocery store), Dreamfields pasta, or very-high fiber whole wheat pasta can be used. Make sure to cook noodles el dente. I've been to Carrabas and brought my own box of Dreamfields pasta. They cooked it for me and put their delicious meat sauce on it. I couldn't tell the difference!
Macaroni and Cheese	Buy a box of Kraft Macaroni & Cheese. Pull out the cheese packet and throw away the noodles. Then, cook one of the low-carb pasta options I mentioned above and prepare as you would a normal Kraft Mac & Cheese dinner.

Oatmeal	Mix one scoop of protein powder with one scoop of Anutra (high fiber product similar to ground flax) blend with ¼ to ½ cup plain yogurt, mix in a tablespoon of olive oil, and add sweetener and cinnamon to taste. We look forward to this almost every morning.
Peanut Butter and Jelly	Make with one slice of lower carb bread –cut in half. Top with peanut butter and sugar free/no sugar added jam.
Ice Cream	Enjoy sugar free/no sugar added ice cream. Edy's is my personal favorite. Perry's is Thin's favorite. If you're craving toppings, try sugar-free fudge, peanut butter, or whipped cream on top.
Smoothie	In a blender, place 1 scoop protein powder, ½ cup yogurt, 4 ice cubes, ¼ - ½ cup berries, ½ cup sugar-free almond milk or soy milk, and add sweetener to taste. Then, blend away ~
Chocolate Dessert	Mix sugar free chocolate pudding with ½ scoop protein powder. Top this with whipped cream.

These examples are intended to show you that, with a little creativity, you can develop a low-carb version of any indulgence. With this knowledge, you will never feel overwhelmed by the diet. There's no reason to. You'll never need to yo-yo diet. Realistically, you may gain a couple of pounds from over indulging on your low-carb treats, but you know that all you need to do to reverse the damage is decrease the carb intake and the weight will come off. We both weigh ourselves nearly every day. Neither of us has allowed our weight to creep up more than three or four pounds since we have reached goal weight.

Support will be a major contributing factor to the success of your diet. A research study from Purdue University showed that women who had supportive partners lost up to 30 percent more weight than those who had no support. We found this to be true in our case. Without Thin, Thinner wouldn't be where she is today, and without Thinner, Thin would not be where she is today. We are each other's sounding board and cheerleader. We keep each other accountable even if it gets annoying. It is worth it because in the end, we look and feel great.

Thin's minister compared our lives with those in a NASCAR race. He explained that in our spiritual walk, we each need a pit crew. He described how a driver could not win the race without his pit crew. The pit crew services the racecar during a pit stop, changing tires, filling the car with gas, and cleaning windshields. Members of the crew also help the driver get around the track as quickly and safely as possible, via radio. The same holds for the low-carb lifestyle. We each need to make sure we have an effective pit crew to support us every step of the way. Finding low carb friends who will share recipes, provide encouragement, and offer fresh solutions is vital to sustaining the motivation needed to go against the grain in the carb-dominated culture in which we live.

A number of low carb websites offer a plethora of free support for those embarking on a low carb lifestyle. Jimmy Moore's Livin' La Vida Low-Carb, Sugar Free Sheila, the Atkins site, George Stella's – Stella Style, Low Carb Luxury, the websites of Drs. Michael and Mary Dan Eades (Protein Power authors), and Dana Carpender's blog are just a few of our favorite sites. There are many other wonderful low carb forums out there, as well. Typing in the words "low carb" into your search engine will bring you to a variety of sites where you will find forums, recipes, and updated research.

Some people need more than just a pep talk to get motivated. Here's a more serious look at how your weight may impact your health. The following is a list of health risks associated with obesity:

- High Blood Pressure
- Diabetes
- Stroke
- Gout
- Arthritis
- Osteoarthritis
- Breast Cancer
- Asthma

- Sleep Apnea
- Gallstones
- Endometrial Cancer
- Cardiovascular Disease
- Gallbladder Disease
- Gynecological Complications
- Urinary Stress Incontinence

Add to all of these a study of 900,000 people in 2003 which concluded that being overweight may be responsible for up to 20 percent of all cancers. Recent studies show a strong correlation between eating carbohydrates and cancer. The findings are showing that carbohydrates feed cancer, and with low carbohydrate diets, cancer may be prevented, and the growth of cancer dramatically decreased, according to a study performed at the British Columbia Cancer Research Center, published on June 14 2011 in the journal "Cancer Research". For Thin and Thinner, this information is motivating enough to keep us on the plan. We also need to remember that the impact of carbohydrates on health does not only affect us, but there are major ramifications for our husbands, children, siblings, parents, and dear friends as well.

Have Faith! Thinner was so enchanted to have come across a study published by Dale Matthews, M.D., author of the Faith Factor. He explained how spiritual practices, such as praying on a regular basis and attending religious services, keep individuals healthier and allow them to live longer, fuller lives. Also, Thin and Thinner pray each day that they can stay committed to a healthy way of eating for the rest of their lives (*Think Thin, Be Thin*).

Keep Busy. When you are busy running around, being productive, and accomplishing things, food is usually the last thing on your mind. When you're bored at home, you know you're going to open the pantry or refrigerator door and just stare, stare, and stare until you see something that'll trigger a craving.

Don't let yourself get too hungry, and don't eat until you're stuffed. Healthy eating requires balance. It is best to eat small, consistent meals throughout the day. This helps keep your metabolism consistently high, and in this way, you are never taking in more food than your body requires for energy. Protein and fat will not be stored as fat in the absence of carbohydrates, but you will not burn excess fat unless you have used up the calories consumed. Also, it is important to stress that if you eat more carbs than will be used up for energy, the remainder gets stored as fat. As a rule of thumb, try waiting 20 minutes before opting for seconds. That is usually how much time your brain needs to process that it has had enough to eat.

Thin and Thinner find that it helps to bring along a snack when running errands all day. This way, we are not tempted to stop for fast food. For example, a little bag of almonds and a mug of hot tea keeps Thinner energized while on-the-go.

Do not rationalize going off the diet, and don't make excuses. People that work long hours often think that they do not have time to eat right or exercise. It is these very same people that will benefit most from a low carb diet with an increase in energy, the ability to think more clearly, and the capacity to be more productive at work. Of course, there is the added benefit of being more attractive. Frankly, in the shallow world of appearances that we are living in today, being overweight is a liability. It may cost you your job or at least a promotion. Unless you are extraordinary at what you do for a living, employers might question your value. If you cannot take care of your own body, they might wonder how you are going to effectively take care of their business.

Be aware. Tell yourself affirmations such as "I know that if I opt for the ice cream made with sugar, I will gain weight. However, if I opt for the sugar-free ice cream, I know that I will not gain weight." Simple, direct thoughts like this will help you to make the right choices for the rest of your life.

Don't forget to eat the most important meal of the day--breakfast! There have been countless studies attesting to this. Those who skip breakfast are four times more likely to suffer from obesity. Breakfast should be your first meal of the day.

Let everyone know that you are following a low-carb lifestyle. In this way you will not be put in an awkward situation where a friend invites you over for spaghetti dinner, or a relative buys you an expensive box of chocolates for your birthday. Also, let everyone know that you do not expect special accommodations. Offer to bring a snack (e.g. celery and dip, cheese platter, or nuts), protein (e.g. shrimp cocktail or deviled eggs), or beverage (e.g. dry white wine) with you if you are not sure of the menu.

Drink water. It helps eliminate toxins and prevents bloating. Some experts recommend drinking specific amounts based on body weight. These quantities may be a bit hard to achieve. Thin and Thinner try to drink as much as they can. They try to be aware of when they are thirsty.

Take supplements as needed. Both Thin and Thinner take various vitamins and minerals to meet their individual dietary needs. It is important to consult your own physician or nutritionist to determine which supplements best support your unique requirements. Start by asking about a good multiple vitamin.

CHAPTER 24: DISPELLING THE MYTHS AND LIES ABOUT THE LOW-CARBOHYDRATE DIET

You may have heard rumors about low-carb dieting or have been mislead in the past about some important truths. Some misguided souls go as far as to nickname it "the bacon and egg diet". The low-carb lifestyle is far from a plate piled high with beef and topped with a large scoop of lard, devoid of any fruits and vegetables. This visual couldn't be further from the truth, and we are going to set the record straight. The following are responses to many low-carb misconceptions.

Low-carb does <u>not</u> mean no-carb. Even on the induction phase of the Atkins Diet, 20 grams of carbohydrates are allowed per day. Thin eats 25 grams of carbs per day, not counting green vegetables. Thinner eats about 40 grams of carbs. Both Thin and Thinner eat significantly more vegetables and berries than they had ever eaten prior to low-carb living.

This diet is <u>not</u> a high protein diet, and it has in no way damaged our kidneys. There has never been a study that showed kidney damage from protein consumption. In fact, recent studies recommend that adults eat meals with at least 30 grams of protein to maintain healthy muscles and bones.

Thin and Thinner usually only have 21 grams per meal and may need to eat more!

Yes, we are eating less food, but we feel much more satisfied and full. This is due to the fact that we are not hungry. Meat is one of the most nutrient rich foods one can eat. Eating adequate amounts of protein, healthy fats, and green vegetables will satisfy our bodies, and as a result, we do not crave more food. Our brains tell us that we are full, and we would literally have to force ourselves to eat after such a meal. Interestingly, we eat more calories in a day than on other diet plans, but instead of gaining weight, we lose weight! There are many good books, mentioned in our bibliography, that explain how protein and fat calories differ from those coming from carbohydrates.

You don't have to give up your pasta forever! You will never eat regular pasta again since this program is a lifestyle, and the plan is meant to be followed for life. But, now there are many low glycemic/low-carb pastas sitting on the shelves of your local grocery store. Thinner's favorite is the "Dreamfields" brand. Family and friends can't tell the difference. Another way to lower the glycemic load of pasta is to cook it al dente. It breaks down much more slowly having less of an impact on blood sugar. But, we enjoy these substitutes sparingly, and rarely when we are above our goal weights. Another option is tofu noodles, often found near the organic foods section of the grocery store. They have the same texture as regular cooked pasta. Once they're rinsed off, dried, and covered with a tasty sauce, we can't tell the difference. Since discovering the Shirataki tofu noodles, Thin exclusively uses them as a pasta substitute. These "noodles" contain only 1 g of net carbs per serving.

Low-carb diets disappeared for a while, but there were extenuating circumstances. Industries that profit from the consumption of refined sugar, flour, and other starchy products formed powerful lobbies which greatly suppressed knowledge regarding the effectiveness and health benefits of low-carb living. You'll find that we have dedicated an entire chapter of this book to the topic. Recent university studies are shedding light on the value of following a low-carbohydrate eating plan.

You might hear, "You're on Atkins? The guy that wrote that book gave himself a heart attack from following his own diet plan." This statement is false. At the age of 72, Dr. Atkins slipped on an icy sidewalk. The impact that the fall had on his head was the cause of his death. It says so on his death certificate.

We do not eat bacon and eggs for breakfast, cheeseburgers sans the bun for lunch, and steak for dinner every night. Though we could do this if we wanted to! Low-carb living is much more exciting than that. For example, a low-carb breakfast might consist of a protein and fruit smoothie or a veggie-filled omelet, lunch might be chicken salad and soup, and for dinner a low-carber might enjoy ahi tuna sashimi or steak teriyaki with roasted vegetables. Snacks can range from small portions of nuts, cheese and fruit, veggies with exciting dips, sugar-free pudding or Jell-O, topped with whipped cream. Mmm… See the meal plan and recipe chapters for more exciting and creative things you can eat.

With this diet, you will get enough nutrients. The simple truth is that you do not need to eat any carbohydrates. According to Drs. Eades and Eades in *The Protein Power Lifeplan*, p. 322, the body can manufacture its own carbohydrates out of fats and protein that we consume. We would be quite healthy on a diet consisting of good sources of protein and fat, along with water and minerals.

Add to this, Thinner's own unscientific study. After consulting with various people who aren't following a low-carb diet, Thinner discovered that most of her friends are not eating nearly the quantity of berries and vegetables that she is, leave alone the essential proteins and healthy fats. She has come to the conclusion that her diet is a much more nutritious alternative to typical American eating habits.

You do not need carbs for energy. In fact, we have found that sugary and starchy carbs actually sap us of our energy. Thin wishes she had known this years ago. At about 3:00 p.m. each afternoon, she would have an energy drain, and be quite lethargic. Realizing that it was time to start cooking dinner, she would eat whatever was available to have enough stamina to prepare the meal. Often, the only convenient ready-to-eat item was a large bag of potato chips. Thin would get through half the bag, and then she could not understand why she felt even more sluggish. She would invariably lie down for about twenty minutes and then force herself to go into the kitchen to cook. She could not understand why the potato chips had let her down. Thin did not know at the time that the carbohydrates were not providing her body with the appropriate fuel. She was essentially putting coal in her gas tank, instead of gasoline, and wondering why her car would not start.

It is not necessary to exercise in order to lose weight on a low-carb diet, but it is strongly recommended. And because the diet restricts carbs, there is a significant weight-loss advantage to working out. Since you are following a low-carb diet, you don't have to work out for as long as everyone else. The rule of thumb is that it takes 20 minutes of cardiovascular exercise before you start burning fat during a workout. That is because in the first 20 minutes of working out, your body is busy burning carbohydrates and sugar as energy before it can get to the fat. This is where low carbers have an advantage. Since we are not storing large amounts of carbohydrates and sugar in our bodies, we go directly into fat burning mode as soon as we start exercising. So, we "low carbers" can get double the workout in half the time! While it takes an average person 40 minutes to get a fat-burning workout, it takes a low-carb dieter only 20 minutes to get the same results!!

Many people reason that because there are websites out there that offer free information and diet plans that warn against low-carb diets, they must have good reasons. This line of reasoning needs to be corrected. Many of these so called "free" sources of diet advice usually are sponsored by companies such as General Mills, Kellogg's, Chex cereal, and other large brand-name companies that rely on selling carb-filled foods as their main source of "dough". And, there are many campaigns going on behind the scenes, purposely giving low-carb eating a bad rap, in order to protect businesses that would implode if the full truth about their products came to light. So, advocates have been hired to make sure that consumers do not stop buying carb-rich and sugar-filled products.

Why Low-Carb Went Away

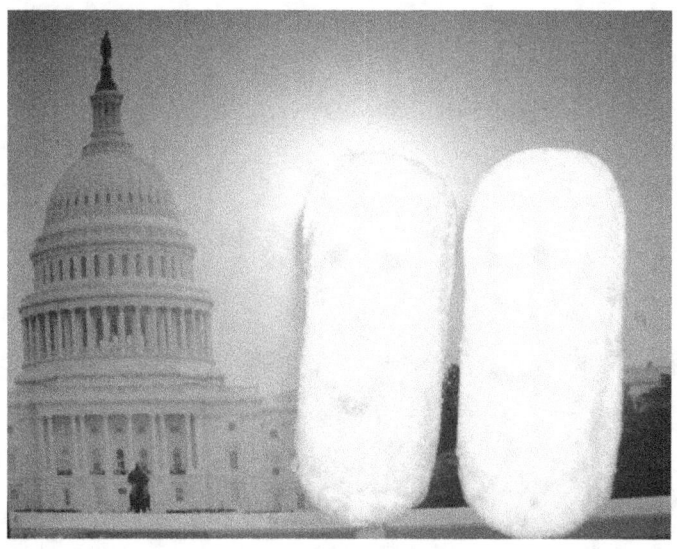

Disclaimer: This illustration is not intended to imply that any particular product influenced any government or private agency to favor carbohydrates in any way. But, it is meant to show that producers of carbohydrate products in general did respond to the low-carb debate.

CHAPTER 25: WHAT WE ARE UP AGAINST

The benefits of following a low-carbohydrate diet became apparent in the first four years of the 21st century. With Dr. Atkins and Drs. Michael and Mary Dan Eades, higher protein, lower-carb programs emerged with huge followings. The effectiveness of this approach to weight loss inspired many to shed dangerous, unhealthy fat. A close friend with type 2 diabetes, while strictly following a low-carb regimen, was instructed by his physician to stop taking insulin. His blood levels were now fine. But then, the tide turned, and low carb diets were seriously questioned. Our friend went off the diet and his diabetic condition returned.

What happened to the low-carb approach? The following headlines will give a good indication of why our government does not endorse low carb diets, why the popularity of low carb diets went away, and why it will be hard to get the truth out.

Drop in wheat consumption worries US Grain Trade

by Carey Gillam
Reuters January 30, 2003
from forum.lowcarber.org1showthread.php?t=83908

Matter of Rising Concern: Waistline and bottom line

As low-carb diets gain in popularity, bakeries are feeling the pinch
by Paul Grimaldi
The Providence Journal   November 13, 2003

Nuts and meat snacks grow

Every type of candy, snack, and confection lost sales in 2003, with the exception of nuts and meat snacks, confirmed by MSA Inc.
by Elliot Maras
Vending Marketwatch.com 2003

Stop dieting?Fat chance!—Declining sales hurt high-carb products

Impact of low carb diets on profits of one of the nation's biggest distributors of rice
by Bill Hensel, Jr.
Houston Chronicle   January 23, 2004

Low-Carb Diets Hit Pizza Biz Hard

by Bob Edwards
NPR   February 4, 2004

Low-Carb Diets Hurt Florida O.J. Sales

Citrus Industry Fights Back with New Health-Drink Ads
by Snigdha Prakash
NPR Morning Edition April 23, 2004

Krispy Kreme is latest victim of low-carb diets

by Paul Nowell, Associated Press
Charlotte, N.C.
USATODAY.com   May 7, 2004

The Trouble with Sugar

"Panorama uncovers remarkable evidence showing the sugar and food lobbies secretly influenced a
major United Nations scientific study into how much
sugar we should be eating"
BBC News October 4, 2004

Low-carb legacy hitting US pasta sales

FOOD navigator.com
November 18, 2004

Wrigley snaps up sweets from Kraft

Kraft decided recently to shed most of its confection
brands, admitting that candy was one of four categories struggling in part because of low-carb diets that
forgo sweets and starchy foods.
by Dave Carpenter
Chicago
Associated Press   November 16, 2004

Bread Industry Biting Back

Using Marketing Campaign As Low-Carb Diets Eat
At Its Bottom Line

by Brian Dakss
New York
The Early Show-CBS News   March 31, 2005

American Diabetes Association peddling nutritional nonsense while accepting money from manufacturer of candy and sodas

Natural News.com
by Jessica Fraser   June 1, 2005

Sugar industry reveals distaste for foes, rivals

The sugar industry attributes recent sugar consumption losses to the popularity of low carb diets.
by Deb Kollars
Sacramento Bee   August 4, 2005

Half-baked

Low-carb dieting prompted a decline in the gelatin/pudding mix segment, cake, cupcake, pie mix, pancake/waffle mixes, cookies, cookie bars, and brownie mixes
by William A. Roberts, Jr.
Prepared Foods Network   May 1, 2006

In a nutshell, it appears evident that low carb diets are bad for the economy and if you follow one, you are un-American. Add to that the countless powerful lobbies that have been at work, influencing authorities from the World Health Organization to the U.S. government in developing the food pyramid.

In an article entitled, "The Ties that Bind," Anthony Colpo, an independent researcher, amassed a huge body of information detailing the extent to which producers of high carbohydrate products have financially influenced private and governmental health organizations.   To read the article, go to

http://www.lowcarportal.com/archives/2004/08/12/the_ties_that_bind.php

The article is originally published in "The Omnivore" (www.theomnivore.com)

Millions of dollars have been and continue to be spent to prevent the truth about low-carb living from being understood by the general public. Ida and Emily owe their lives and good health to Dr. Atkins, The Eades, and many others who have persevered in getting the message out about the health benefits of limiting carbohydrate consumption. We have written this book to share what we have learned in the hopes that in some way this information will help to improve the quality of life for others.

CHAPTER 26: TOOLS

- Please feel free to photocopy the following pages.
- Make multiple copies of the grocery list to use for weekly shopping excursions. Run it back-to-back if possible. Just check off the items needed for that week.
- The journal page will be particularly helpful to those who are just starting out. For the first 6 months, we wrote down everything we ate in order to learn the carb counts and to make sure we were consuming enough protein.

Low-Carb Journal

Checklist: Date: _____

- ☐ I limited my net carbs to 25 grams
  (excluding carbs in green vegetables) today.
- ☐ I ate a sufficient amount of protein today,
  about 21 g per meal or a minimum of
  63 g for the day. along with non-starchy
  vegetables, and healthy fats.
- ☐ I exercised for at least 25 minutes today
  (5 days per week) for accelerated weight
  loss.

Daily Food Plan:

	Total Net Carbs

Breakfast

	____ g

Lunch

	____ g

Dinner

<pre>
_____
_____
_____   ____g
_____
_____
</pre>

Snacks (2 per day)

<pre>
_____
_____
_____   ____g
_____
_____
</pre>

Daily Carb Total: _____g

Low-Carb Lifestyle Grocery List

Meat, Deli, and Fish Departments

- ☐ ground beef
- ☐ beef tenderloins
- ☐ sirloin steaks
- ☐ thin sliced sirloin steaks
- ☐ roast beef
- ☐ prime rib
- ☐ beef riblets
- ☐ any other beef cut
- ☐ tilapia
- ☐ lump crab (not imitation!)
- ☐ shrimp
- ☐ sea bass
- ☐ grouper
- ☐ salmon
- ☐ filet of sole
- ☐ chicken cutlets
- ☐ chicken breasts with bones
- ☐ boneless chicken breasts
- ☐ pork riblets
- ☐ pork tenderloin
- ☐ breakfast pork sausages (pork, chicken, or turkey)

- ☐ Italian sausage (pork, chicken, or turkey)
- ☐ baby back pork ribs
- ☐ Canadian bacon
- ☐ bacon
- ☐ ham
- ☐ turkey
- ☐ lamb
- ☐ pepperoni
- ☐ veal cutlets
- ☐ other meats _____

Cheese and Egg Departments

- ☐ eggs
- ☐ shredded parmesan cheese
- ☐ shredded Romano cheese
- ☐ Monterey Jack (sliced, shredded, and cubes)
- ☐ Mozzarella (sliced, shredded, and cubes)
- ☐ Cheddar (sliced, shredded, and cubes)
- ☐ Provolone cheese
- ☐ string cheese
- ☐ *The Kitchen Table Bakers Hand Made Gourmet Wafer Crisps*

Produce Department

- ☐ artichoke hearts (fresh or frozen)
- ☐ asparagus
- ☐ avocadoes
- ☐ broccoli (fresh or frozen)
- ☐ brussel sprouts
- ☐ carrots (limited use)
- ☐ cauliflower (fresh or frozen)
- ☐ celery
- ☐ cucumbers
- ☐ eggplant
- ☐ garlic
- ☐ lettuce (Romaine and other salad greens)
- ☐ mushrooms
- ☐ green onions
- ☐ white onions
- ☐ shallots
- ☐ peppers
- ☐ spinach
- ☐ spaghetti squash
- ☐ string beans (fresh or frozen)
- ☐ summer squash
- ☐ tomatoes
- ☐ zucchini squash
- ☐ water chestnuts
- ☐ other green vegetables

_____

- ☐ strawberries
- ☐ blueberries
- ☐ raspberries
- ☐ blackberries
- ☐ lemons

Dairy Aisle

- ☐ Half and Half
- ☐ butter
- ☐ cream
- ☐ sour cream
- ☐ whipped cream
- ☐ yogurt, plain or sugar-free (Dannon Carb-
- ☐ Control vanilla is fine)
- ☐ cream cheese

Health Food Aisle

- ☐ almond butter
- ☐ almond flour
- ☐ ground flaxseed or Anutra
- ☐ low-carb crackers
- ☐ Shirataki Tofu noodles
- ☐ soy milk (no sugar added)
- ☐ Stevia liquid
- ☐ Stevia packets
- ☐ Guar Gum
- ☐ Thick N' Thin—Not Starch
- ☐ Xanthan gum

- ☐ unsweetened protein powder (approx. 21
- ☐ grams of protein per serving)
- ☐ flax chips

Interior Aisles:

Fat:
- ☐ olive oil
- ☐ canola oil
- ☐ any other healthy oil (no transfats)
- ☐ mayonnaise
- ☐ olive oil spray
- ☐ salad dressing (with 2 carbs or less per serving)

Nuts and Seeds:
- ☐ almonds (whole)
- ☐ almonds (sliced)
- ☐ macadamia nuts
- ☐ peanuts
- ☐ pecans
- ☐ pistachios
- ☐ sunflower seeds
- ☐ walnuts

Sugar Free Treats and Snacks(with no more than 12 net carbs per serving):
- ☐ sugar-free candy
- ☐ no sugar added ice cream

- ☐ sugar-free jello
- ☐ sugar-free popsicles
- ☐ sugar-free pudding
- ☐ sugar-free cookies
- ☐ low-carb protein bar

Other items:
- ☐ apple cider vinegar
- ☐ barbecue sauce (12 g net carbs or less per serving)
- ☐ beef broth
- ☐ cocoa powder (unsweetened)
- ☐ chicken bouillon
- ☐ chicken broth
- ☐ flour (regular—for thickening sauces and gravies)
- ☐ Ghiradelli 100 % Cacao or other unsweetened chocolate chips for baking
- ☐ green olives
- ☐ hot sauce
- ☐ mustard
- ☐ olives (black)
- ☐ olives (green)
- ☐ peanut butter (creamy or crunchy)
- ☐ soy sauce
- ☐ tomato juice
- ☐ tomato paste
- ☐ tomato puree

- ☐ tomato sauce
- ☐ Truvia packets
- ☐ white vinegar
- ☐ Worcestershire sauce

Spices:
- ☐ basil
- ☐ black pepper
- ☐ cayenne (red) pepper
- ☐ chili powder
- ☐ cinnamon
- ☐ garlic salt
- ☐ oregano
- ☐ parsley
- ☐ rosemary
- ☐ salt

- ☐ vanilla
- ☐ white pepper

Beverages:
- ☐ coffee
- ☐ tea
- ☐ water
- ☐ unsweetened iced tea
- ☐ diet cola (sweetened with Splenda—not aspartame)
- ☐ sugar free drinks
- ☐ dry wine, red or white
- ☐ non-sweet liquor

_____

- ☐ Miller Lite beer or other low-carb beer

REFERENCES

The Science Behind the Diet:

Atkins, Robert C. *Dr. Atkins' New Diet Revolution*. New York: Avon Books, 2002.

Eades, Michael R. and Mary Dan Eades. *The Protein Power Lifeplan*. New York: Warner Books, Inc., 2000.

Taubes, Gary. *Good Calories, Bad Calories*. New York: Random House, Inc., 2007.

Taubes, Gary. *Why we Get Fat and What to Do About It*. New York: Alfred A. Knopf., 2011.

Westman, Dr. Eric, Dr. Stephen D. Phinney, and Dr. Jeff S. Volek. *New Atkins for a New You*. New York: Simon and Schuster, Inc., 2010.

Thin's Journey to Maintain a Healthy Weight:

Allan, Christian B. and Wolfgang Lutz. *Life Without Bread: How a Low-Carbohydrate Diet Can Save Your Life*. Chicago: Keats Publishing, 2000.

Atkins, Robert C. *Dr. Atkins' New Diet Revolution*. New York: Avon Books, 2002.

Appleton, Nancy. *Lick the Sugar Habit.* Garden City Park, New York: Avery Publishing Group, 1996.

Eades, Michael R. and Mary Dan Eades. *The Protein Power Lifeplan.* New York: Warner Books, Inc., 2000.

Schwarzbein, Diana and Nancy Deville. *The Schwarzbein Principle.* Deerfield Beach, Florida: Health Communications, Inc., 1999.

How the Diet Has Changed Thin's Life:

Layman, Donald K. "Dietary Guidelines Should Reflect New Understandings About Adult Protein Needs." Department of Food Science and Human Nutrition, University of Illinois, Urbana, March 13, 2009 (www.nutritionandme-tabolism.com/content/ 6/1/12).

"Causes of Brain Fog and Ways to Resolve It," http//www.avianweb.com/memoryloss.html, 2006

Bennett, Connie, Stephen Sinatra, and Nicholas Perricone (Foreword by). Sugar Shock!: How Sweets and Simple Carbs Can Derail Your Life-and How You Can Get Back on Track. USA: Penguin Group, 2006

Amen, Daniel G. "Optimizing Brain Function." *Brain and Mind Magazine,* December 31, 2002.

Exercise—Thinner Used to Get Tired Just Thinking About It:

Atkins, Robert C. *Dr. Atkins' New Diet Revolution*. New York: Avon Books, 2002, pp. 142, 287 – 288.

Atkins, Robert C. *Atkins for Life*. New York: St. Martin's Press, 2003, p. 85.

Thinner's Advice on How to Satisfy Your Sweet Tooth Without Going Off the Diet:

Johnny Bowden. *Living the Low Carb Life*. New York: Sterling Publishing Co., Inc., 2004, p. 228.

"High Fructose Corn Syrup,"http://www.solarnavigator.net/solar_cola/high_fructose_corn_syrup.htm

Thinner's Thoughts on Constipation and Elimination:

Leong, Kristie, M.D. "What Are the Dangers of Laxative Abuse?". healthmad.com/health/what-are-the-dangers-of-laxative-abuse/, May 23, 2009.

Emily's physician in Lakewood Ranch, Florida

"EGCG Review," www.dietspotlight.com/egcg-review/

Tips to Stay Motivated and Continue Low-Carbing for Life:

Helmering, Doris Wild and Dianne Hales. *Think Thin, Be Thin*. New York: Broadway Books, 2005, pp. 17, 53, 66, 67, 148, and 192.

"Weight Loss: Health Risks Associated with Obesity," http://www.webmd.com/cholesterol-management/obesity-health-risks, 2009.

Calle, Eugenia, et al. "Overweight, Obesity, and Mortality from Cancer in a Prospectively Studied Cohort of U.S. Adults," New England Journal of Medicine 348, no 17 (April 24, 2003): I625.

The Myths and Lies About the Low-Carbohydrate Diet:

Johnny Bowden. *Living the Low Carb Life*. New York: Sterling Publishing Co., Inc., 2004, pp. 67 and 198.

Eades, Michael R. and Mary Dan Eades. *The Protein Power Lifeplan*. New York: Warner Books, Inc., 2000, pp. 9 and 322.

http://www.chex.com/products/products.aspx

http://www.generalmills.com/corporate/health_wellness/index.aspx

http://www.kelloggs.com/nutrition/

"What Was the Cause of Robert Atkins' Death?" http://answers.yahoo.com/question/index?qid=2008010518343AAXBKIo

"Why Has My Low Carb Diet Stopped Working?" http://lowcarbeating.com/low-carb help/why-has-my-low-carb-diet-stopped-working , 2003.

What We Are Up Against:

Gillman, Carey. "Drop in Wheat Consumption Worries US Grain Trade." *Reuters*, January 30, 2003 from forum.lowcarber.org1showthread.php?t=83908.

Grimaldi, Paul. "Matter of Rising Concern: Waistline and Bottom Line." *The Providence Journal*, November 13, 2003.

Maras, Elliot. "Nuts and Meat Snacks Grow." *Vending Marketwatch*.com, 2003.

Hensel, Bill, Jr. "Stop Dieting? Fat Chance!— Declining Sales Hurt High-Carb Products." *Houston Chronicle*, January 23, 2004.

Edwards, Bob. "Low-Carb Diets Hit Pizza Biz Hard." *NPR*, February 4, 2004.

Prakash, Snigdha. "Low-Carb Diets Hurt Florida O.J. Sales." *NPR Morning Edition*, April 23, 2004.

Nowell, Paul. "Krispy Kreme is Latest Victim of Low-Carb Diets." *USATODAY.com*, May 7, 2004.

"The Trouble with Sugar." *BBC News*, October 4, 2004.

"Low-Carb Legacy Hitting US Pasta Sales." *FOOD navigator.com*, November 18, 2004.

Carpenter, Dave. "Wrigley Snaps up Sweets from Kraft." *Associated Press*, November 16, 2004.

Dakss, Brian. "Bread Industry Biting Back." *The Early Show-CBS News*, March 31, 2005.

Fraser, Jessica. "American Diabetes Association Peddling Nutritional Nonsense While Accepting Money from Manufacturer of Candy and Sodas." *Natural News.com*, June 1, 2005.

Kollars, Deb. "Sugar Industry Reveals Distaste for Foes, Rivals." *Sacramento Bee*, August 4, 2005

Roberts, William A., Jr. "Half-Baked." *Prepared Foods Network*, May 1, 2006.

Colpo, Anthony. "The Ties that Bind." The Omnivore, August 12, 2004 (www.theomnivore.com).

In order to maintain a healthy low-carb lifestyle, we strongly recommend reading a variety of books on the subject. Following this advice will assist you in staying focused, motivated, and informed. Here is a list of books that have guided us along our low-carb journey–educating us, inspiring us, and giving us hope, motivation, and new ideas every day.

BIBLIOGRAPHY

Allan, Christian B. and Wolfgang Lutz. *Life Without Bread: How a Low-Carbohydrate Diet Can Save Your Life.* Chicago: Keats Publishing, 2000.

Appleton, Nancy. *Lick the Sugar Habit.* Garden City Park, New York: Avery Publishing Group, 1996.

Atkins Health and Medical Information Services. *The Atkins Essentials.* New York: Avon Books, 2004

Atkins, Robert C. *Atkins for Life.* New York: St. Martin's Press, 2003.

Atkins, Robert C. *Dr. Atkins' New Diet Revolution.* New York: Avon Books, 2002.

Bowden, Jonny. *Living the Low Carb Life.* New York: Sterling Publishing Co., Inc., 2004.

Carpender, Dana. *How I Gave Up My Low-Fat Diet and Lost 40 Pounds...and How You Can Too!* Gloucester, Massachusetts: Fair Winds Press, 2003.

D'Adamo, Peter J. with Catherine Whitney. *Blood Type O: Food, Beverage, and Supplement Lists from Eat Right 4 Your Type.* New York: The Berkley Publishing Group, 2002.

D'Adamo, Peter J. with Catherine Whitney. *Eat Right 4 Your Type.* New York: G.P.Putnam's Sons, 1996.

Eades, Michael R. and Mary Dan Eades. *The Protein Power Lifeplan.* New York: Warner Books, Inc., 2000.

Eades, Michael R. and Mary Dan Eades. *The 30-Day Low-Carb Diet Solution.* Hoboken, New Jersey: John Wiley and Sons, Inc., 2003.

Helmering, Doris Wild and Dianne Hales. *Think Thin, Be Thin.* New York: Broadway Books, 2005.

Northrup, Christiane. *The Wisdom of Menopause.* New York: Bantam Dell, 2006.

Pescatore, Fred. *Thin for Good. New York*: John Wiley and Sons, Inc., 2000.

Schwarzbein, Diana and Nancy Deville. *The Schwarzbein Principle.* Deerfield Beach, Florida: Health Communications, Inc., 1999.

Taubes, Gary. *Good Calories, Bad Calories.* New York: Random House, Inc., 2007.

Taubes, Gary. *Why we Get Fat and What to Do About It.* New York: Alfred A. Knopf., 2011.

Trager, Stuart L. and Colette Heimowitz. *The All-New Atkins Advantage.* New York: St. Martin's Press, 2007.

Westman, Dr. Eric, Dr. Stephen D. Phinney, and Dr. Jeff S. Volek. *New Atkins for a New You.* New York: Simon and Schuster, Inc., 2010.

Recipes

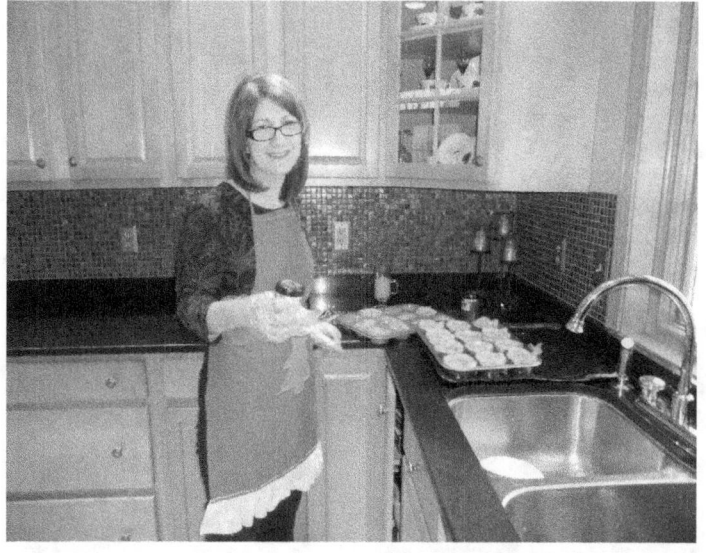

On the pages that follow, you will find delicious
recipes such as Ham and Egg Cups.

Vegetables

Note: If the recipe contains carbs from any source other than non-starchy vegetables, the carb count is noted. If the recipe does not note the carb count, it is insignificant.

Roasted Vegetables

Ingredients:

fresh produce:
- asparagus
- string beans
- broccoli
- cauliflower
- mushrooms

spices: salt, pepper, and garlic salt

2 tbsp. olive oil

Directions:

Wash and dry any of the above vegetables.
Line a large flat pan with parchment paper.
Mix oil with vegetables, arranging vegetables in a single layer in pan.
Sprinkle lightly with spices.
Bake at 400 degrees for 35 minutes.

Variations:

- After roasting, add fresh squeezed lemon.
- After roasting, sprinkle with grated parmesan cheese.
- Drizzle with Kitchen Bouquet and Montreal Seasoning before roasting.
- Dot with butter before roasting.

Tips:

To save time, buy the packaged vegetables that are pre-washed and cut in the produce department.

If other items are in the oven at a different temperature, adjust as below:

- 350 degrees for 45 minutes
- 375 degrees for 40 minutes
- 425 degrees for 30 minutes (use foil instead of parchment paper)
- 450 degrees for 25 minutes (use foil instead of parchment paper)

Note:

Don't concern yourself with the carb count on this recipe. All of these are non-starchy vegetables with fiber.

Sautéed Broccoli

Ingredients:

1 lb. bag of broccoli florets (pre-washed)
1 tsp. salt
2 large cloves of garlic (sliced thin)
2 tbsp. olive oil
1 tbsp. butter
½ tsp. salt
¼ tsp. pepper

Directions:

Rinse florets.
Cover and boil for 15 minutes in salted water.
Drain well.
Sauté garlic in olive oil and butter.
Add broccoli, salt, and pepper.
Cook for 1 minute.

Note:

Serves 4

Mashed Cauliflower (Mock Mashed Potatoes)

Ingredients:

2 heads cauliflower separated into florets (8 cups cooked cauliflower)*
8 tbsp. butter (1 stick–melted)
1 tsp. salt
¼ tsp. white pepper
16 oz. carton of sour cream
12 oz. sharp cheddar, shredded (3 cups)
12 slices of cooked chopped bacon (optional)

Directions:

Boil cauliflower in salted water for 25 minutes or until tender.
Drain cooked cauliflower very well.
Combine remaining ingredients (except bacon).
Puree in food processor.
Fold in bacon.
Bake uncovered in a 9 by 13 inch pan at 350 degrees for 30 min.

Notes:

12 servings

The sour cream adds about 2 carbs per serving to the non-starchy vegetables.

For parties, this recipe can be prepared (unbaked) the day before and refrigerated in a plastic bowl.

Bake the next day in a 9 by 13 inch pan at 350 degrees for 45 minutes.

5 bags of frozen cauliflower can be substituted for the fresh produce. The results are good, but not quite as spectacular.

This is a great side for Thanksgiving dinner.

<u>Variations:</u>

Add 16 oz. of cream cheese and 4 green onions. The cream cheese adds an additional carb per serving.

* Use 5 bags of prewashed and cut cauliflower to save time.

Sautéed Green Beans

Ingredients:

1 ½ lbs. of pre-washed green beans
1 tsp. salt
4 large cloves of garlic (sliced thin)
2 tbsp. olive oil
1 tbsp. butter
½ tsp. salt
¼ tsp. pepper

Directions:

Remove ends.
Rinse green beans.
Cover and boil for 25 minutes in salted water.
Drain well.
Sauté garlic in olive oil and butter.
Add green beans, salt, and pepper.
Stir and sauté for 1 minute.

Note:

Serves 4

Asian Style Spinach

Ingredients:

1 pound bag of baby spinach
2 tbsp. olive oil
1 tbsp. soy sauce

Directions:

Wash and dry spinach.
In electric skillet or large frying pan, heat olive oil.
Add spinach.
Cover and cook for 2 minutes.
Add soy sauce.
Remove cover and cook until excess liquid is gone.

Note:

Serves 3

The spinach will seem like a very small portion when it is cooked.

Spinach Bars

<u>Ingredients:</u>

1 lb. bag of frozen spinach
2 eggs
1 cup heavy cream
spices:
- ½ tsp. salt
- ¼ tsp. pepper
- ¼ tsp. garlic powder

¼ cup of chopped onion
2 tbsp. olive oil
4 tbsp. butter
1 cup of shredded cheddar cheese

<u>Directions:</u>

Thaw spinach, drain, and squeeze out excess liquid.
Set aside.
Grease an 8 inch square pan. Set aside.
Wisk eggs with cream and spices. Set aside.

Sauté onions in olive oil.
Add spinach to frying pan.
Continue cooking for 3 minutes.
Add 2 tbsp. butter to melt.
Pour spinach mixture into egg mixture.
Stir in cheese.
Pour into square baking pan.
Dot with the remaining butter.
Bake uncovered for 30 minutes at 375 degrees.

Wait 10 minutes. Then, cut into 8 bars.

Note:

8 servings

The cream and onion add about 1 gram net carb per serving to the non-starchy vegetables.

Zucchini Hash browns

<u>Ingredients:</u>

3 cups of grated zucchini (A grating tool on the food processor works well!)
1 tsp. salt
2 beaten eggs
½ cup of grated parmesan cheese
¼ cup chopped onion
¼ tsp. salt
¼ tsp. pepper
2 tbsp. flour
2 tbsp. olive oil
2 tbsp. butter

<u>Directions:</u>

Combine grated zucchini with 1 tsp. of salt and place in colander.

Set the colander above a bowl and press zucchini to squeeze out as much moisture as possible or twist it in a clean cheese cloth.

Grated zucchini can be stored in the refrigerator for 2 days. So, it could be grated a few days in advance. This dries the zucchini nicely!

The zucchini must be very dry or it will never brown. Blend drained (dried) zucchini with eggs, cheese, onion, salt, pepper, and flour.

Use ¼ cup of zucchini mixture to form mounds.

Set frying pan or electric skillet to medium-high heat.

Add olive oil and butter to pan.

Sauté zucchini mounds, flattening to shape into patties.

Cook about 3 minutes per side, until golden brown and cooked through.

Then, break apart with spatula and continue to brown for a few more minutes.

Notes:

4 servings

Each serving contains about 4 grams net carbs.

Zucchini - Bacon Stir Fry

<u>Ingredients:</u>

2.2 ounce package of nitrate free bacon
1 medium zucchini
2 heaping tbsp. grated parmesan cheese
¼ tsp. dried thyme leaves
Dash of pepper

<u>Directions:</u>

Pre-cook bacon in skillet on medium heat and drain fat.

Slice zucchini into ¼ inch rounds, add to pan with bacon, and continue to cook over medium to high heat until zucchini and bacon are browned and cooked to your desired level of crunchiness.

Add parmesan, thyme, and pepper.

<u>Notes:</u>

Makes several side dish servings or 1 large serving

5 grams net carbs per serving

Dinner Salad

<u>Ingredients:</u>

Romaine lettuce
chopped white or Vidalia onions
sliced green onions
sliced cucumbers
chopped tomatoes with seeds removed
jumbo green olives (sliced)
shredded cheese (cheddar or blend)
sliced almonds
Good Seasons Mild Italian Dressing

<u>Directions:</u>

Wash and dry lettuce.
Add any or all of the other items.
Serve dressing on the side.

Main Dishes

Meat Sauce with Tofu Noodles

Ingredients:

1 lb. of ground beef
½ tsp. salt
¼ tsp. pepper
2 cups tomato sauce (from 24 oz. jar of Chef's pasta sauce) or other tomato sauce
2 pkgs. Shirataki Tofu noodles
shredded Romano cheese

Directions:

Sauté ground beef in sauce pan. Drain excess fat.
Add salt and pepper.
Reduce heat, add sauce, and continue cooking for 20 min.
Rinse tofu noodles well. Drain in a strainer and pat dry with paper towels.
Microwave noodles for 2 minutes. Pat dry again.
Top noodles with meat sauce.
Sprinkle with cheese.

Note:

Makes 4 servings

12 grams net carbs per serving

Grilled Filet Mignon

<u>Ingredients:</u>

2 pounds of beef tenderloin filets (about 1 ¼ inch thick)
olive oil for basting*
salt
pepper
garlic salt

<u>Directions:</u>

Set the grill to high.
Coat the filets in oil.
Brush oil onto the grill grates.
On a very hot grill, sear the filets for about 1 minute per side.
Continue to grill approximately 5 minutes more per side, seasoning with salt, pepper, and garlic salt.

<u>Notes:</u>

Makes 5 (6 oz.) servings

Steaks will be medium. For medium-well, add 2 minutes of cooking time per side. For medium-rare, grill 4 minutes per side.

* We use Wegman's basting oil.

Beef Vegetable Soup

Ingredients:

1 ½ pounds sirloin steak (or organic strip steaks)
1 ½ cup of chopped onion
3 5.5-ounce cans tomato juice
1 6-ounce can tomato paste
seasonings:
- 2 tsp. salt
- 1 tsp. pepper
- 1 tsp. dried parsley
- 1 tbsp. Worcestershire sauce
- ½ tsp. chili powder

4 cups of beef broth (or a 26 oz. can of beef stock)
2 cups of water
vegetables:
- 1 cup of chopped or sliced celery
- 2 medium carrots, chopped or sliced
- 1 cup chopped fresh mushrooms
- 2 cups of frozen cut green beans or 2 cups of fresh zucchini cut into cubes.

Directions:

Trim fat off steaks.
In large stock pot, brown steak (both sides) and onion in a little olive oil.
Add tomato juice, tomato paste, seasoning, broth, and water.
Cover and simmer for 2 hours.

Remove the meat and cut into cubes.

Return meat to pot and add the remaining vegetables.*

Cover and simmer for 1 more hour.

Notes:

Makes 8 servings.

7 grams net carbs per serving

Add zucchini for the last 30 minutes of cooking.

Teriyaki Skirt Steak

Ingredients:

1 1/2 pounds skirt steak
2 green onions, finely chopped
4 garlic cloves, pushed through a press
3 tbsp reduced sodium soy sauce
1 tbsp sesame oil
¼ cup white wine
2 packets of Splenda
2 tbsp dry toasted sesame seeds

Directions:

Place all ingredients in a bowl or plastic bag to marinate.

Refrigerate 1 hour, turning meat periodically.

Preheat grill or prepare skillet over medium-high heat.

Remove meat from marinade; discard marinade. Grill or sauté steak 3 to 4 minutes per side for medium doneness.

Notes:

Makes 4 servings

4 grams net carbs per serving

Super Charged Beef or Chicken Taco's

Ingredients:

½ white onion
1 medium zucchini
1 red pepper
2 cloves of garlic
1 tbsp. olive oil
1 packet taco seasoning
1 pound ground beef or chicken
Low carb wraps

toppings:

- shredded cheese
- diced tomato
- guacamole
- sour cream
- salsa
- lettuce

Directions:

Dice vegetables and sauté in olive oil in large pot until vegetables are soft.

Add beef or shredded chicken, cook until browned.

Mix in taco seasoning.

Serve with toppings, on low carb wraps, or over lettuce.

Notes:

Makes 4 servings

Contains approx. 5 net carbs without wraps.

Chicken Noodle Soup

Ingredients:

2 pkgs. miropox (chopped celery, carrots, and onions—from produce aisle) (or ½ cup of each)
1 package of chopped onion (or 1 medium onion chopped)
1 large zucchini (cubed)
4 tbsp. butter
1 pound boneless, skinless chicken breasts or thighs
seasonings:

- ½ tsp pepper
- 1 tsp. salt
- 1 tsp. dried parsley
- 1/8 tsp. garlic salt
- 1 package of Knorr Vegetable Soup Mix or

4 cans (14 oz.) chicken broth
3 pkgs. of Shirataki Tofu noodles
Romano cheese

Directions:

Sauté miropox and onions in butter until vegetables are soft.
Add chicken and seasonings. Cover and cook for 20 minutes.
Add chicken broth and chopped zucchini. Cover and simmer for another 30 minutes.
Remove chicken. Cut chicken into small pieces.
Add chicken back into broth.

Rinse Shirataki tofu noodles well. Drain in strainer and dry with paper towels. Microwave tofu noodles for 2 minutes. Place in soup bowls.

Top noodles with chicken soup. Sprinkle with grated Romano cheese.

Note:

8 servings

5 grams net carbs per serving

Almond-Crusted Chicken Tenders

Ingredients

6 tablespoons of melted butter
3 large boneless, skinless chicken breasts, each cut into 3 long strips
½ cup grated Parmesan cheese
1 cup of almond flour or ground almonds
½ tsp. salt
½ tsp. ground red pepper (cayenne)
½ tsp. dried parsley

Directions:

Mix Parmesan cheese, almond flour, salt, ground red pepper, and parsley. Set aside.
Melt butter in microwave.
Dip chicken pieces in melted butter.
Then, dip chicken in flour mixture.
Place chicken on a large pan lined with parchment paper.
Bake uncovered in oven for 35 minutes at 375 degrees.

Notes:

Makes 4 servings

1.5 grams net carbs per serving

Barbecued Chicken

Ingredients:

4 small bone-in split chicken breasts
seasonings:
- salt
- pepper
- garlic salt

barbecue sauce (12 carbs or fewer per serving)

Directions:

Par boil chicken breasts for 20 minutes in a pot on the stove.

Turn stove off and allow chicken to rest in the pot for an additional 30 minutes.

Place chicken breasts on <u>hot</u> grill. Add seasonings to both sides.

Add barbecue sauce to top.

After 5 minutes, turn chicken and baste with barbecue sauce.

Grill another 5 minutes.

Notes:

4 servings

Barbecue sauce will add carbs. Count the number of carbs per serving in your daily carb total.

A recipe for barbecue sauce is in the back if you wish to use it.

Nona's Chicken in Spicy Sauce (Chicken Pizziola)

Ingredients:

½ cup onion (chopped)
3 large cloves of garlic
6 boneless chicken breasts (about 3 lbs.)
salt and pepper
¾ cup of Chablis
1 and ½ tbsp. apple cider vinegar (or white vinegar)
3 tsp. sugar (or 3 packets of Truvia)
¼ tsp. of the following spices:
  • parsley

  • oregano

  • basil

  • rosemary
1 can of tomato puree (29 oz.)
½ cup chicken broth
1 and ½ tsp. salt
½ tsp. pepper
olive oil (extra light tasting) (enough to barely coat bottom of pan)

Directions:

Sauté' onion and 1 minced clove of garlic in olive oil. Set aside.
Coat bottom of a large casserole pan with oil.
Add chicken in one layer. Turn Chicken to coat.
Sprinkle with salt and pepper.
Spread sautéed onions and garlic on chicken.
Cover and bake at 450 degrees for 30 minutes.

In large kettle, mix together the following:
- wine
- 2 remaining cloves of minced garlic
- vinegar
- sugar
- 4 spices
- tomato puree
- chicken broth
- 1 and ½ tsp. salt
- ½ tsp. pepper

Add sauce to chicken. Cover with foil.
Reduce oven to 350 degrees and continue baking for 1 ½ hours.

<u>Notes:</u>

Makes 6 servings
Serve with rice for the non-low-carbers and with tofu noodles for the low-carbers.

Each serving with ½ package (4 oz.) of Tofu Shirataki contains about 9 net carbs.
(The tofu noodles have 1 net carb.)

Roast Chicken Breasts with Cheese Sauce

<u>Ingredients:</u>

3 pounds of chicken breasts (on bones) with skin
2 tbsp. butter
1 tsp. salt
½ tsp pepper
½ tsp. garlic salt

<u>Directions:</u>

Wash and dry chicken breasts. Remove skin.
Top chicken with salt, pepper, and garlic salt.
Dot with butter. Replace skin.
Roast chicken for 50 minutes in oven at 375 degrees.

Serve with cheese sauce. (See recipe in this book.)

<u>Note:</u>

Makes 4 servings

Cheese Sauce

<u>Ingredients:</u>

3 tbsps. melted butter
2 cups shredded sharp cheddar cheese
1 cup sour cream
¼ tsp. salt
¼ tsp black pepper
¼ tsp. cayenne pepper (red pepper)
1 tsp. dried parsley

<u>Directions:</u>

Heat all ingredients in a pan until melted.

<u>Note:</u>

Makes 8 servings

2 grams net carbs per serving

Fast and Delicious Chicken in Cheese Sauce

Ingredients:

¾ cup half and half
3 tbsps. melted butter
2 cups shredded sharp cheddar cheese
½ cup sour cream
½ tsp. salt
¼ tsp white pepper
½ tsp. dried parsley

Directions:

Boil 2 pounds of organic chicken breasts for 30 minutes.
Remove from water and break apart.

Heat and stir together:

¾ cup of half and half
3 tblsp. butter

Add:

½ cup sour cream
2 cups shredded sharp cheddar
½ tsp. salt
¼ tsp. white pepper
½ tsp. dried parsley

Stir chicken into cheese sauce and serve.

<u>Note:</u>

Makes 8 servings

2 grams net carbs per serving

Perfect Burgers on the Grill

<u>Ingredients:</u>

1 pound 95 % lean ground beef
1 tsp. salt
¼ tsp. cayenne pepper (red pepper)
¼ tsp. garlic salt

<u>Directions:</u>

Mix (knead) all ingredients together using plastic food gloves.
Divide into 4 patties.
Brush with soy sauce while grilling.

<u>Note:</u>

Makes 4 servings

2 grams net carbs per serving
Serve between 2 cheese wraps. (See recipe)

No Carb Cheese Wraps

(Perfect rolls for hot dogs, hamburgers, or sausages!)

Ingredients:

4 oz. block of cheddar cheese
1 egg
1 tblsp. olive oil

Directions:

Break apart and melt 4 oz. cheddar cheese in micro-wave. (about 45 seconds)
Mix melted cheese with 1 egg.
Heat 1 tblsp. of olive oil in a small non-stick pan on high.
Add 1/3 of cheese mixture. Spread so that it thinly covers the bottom of the pan.
Heat on high until it is golden brown.
Carefully flip and lightly brown the other side.
Place on wax paper, and make the next wrap.

These are delicious wrapped around a hot dog or a sausage. Use 2 small ones for a hamburger.

Note:

Makes 3 wraps

Roasted Barbecued Pork Tenderloin

Ingredients:

2 pork tenderloins (about 2 pounds)
barbecue sauce (with 12 carbs or less per serving)
foil pan or aluminum foil
4 tbsp. olive oil (approx.)
salt, pepper, and garlic powder

Directions:

Preheat oven to 450 degrees.
In foil lined pan, coat tenderloins in olive oil.
Shake on salt, pepper, and garlic powder.
Place uncovered in oven for 35 minutes.
After 20 minutes, slather on barbecue sauce.
Continue roasting for another 15 minutes.
Remove tenderloins from oven and cover with foil for 15 minutes.

Note:

Serves 6

Barbecue sauce will add carbs. Count the number of carbs per serving in your daily carb total.

Barbecue Ribs All Year

Ingredients:

3 pounds of pork or beef riblets (or 2 racks of baby back ribs)
barbecue sauce (12 or fewer carbs per serving)

Directions:

Place ribs in a foil lined pan.
Bake uncovered for 2 hours at 275 degrees.
Brush top side with barbecue sauce.
Bake for 30 more minutes.
Turn racks of ribs over and brush with barbecue sauce.
Increase temperature to 375 degrees and bake for another 30 minutes.

Note:

Serves 4

Count the number of carbs per serving in your daily carb total.

Almond-Crusted Tilapia

<u>Ingredients</u>

2 slightly beaten eggs
2 pounds of tilapia filets
¼ cup grated Parmesan cheese
½ cup of almond flour or ground almonds
½ tsp. salt
¼ tsp. pepper
1 tbsp. fresh chopped parsley
1 lemon

<u>Directions:</u>

Mix Parmesan cheese, almond flour, salt, and pepper, and parsley. Set aside.
Dip tilapia pieces in eggs.
Then, dip tilapia in flour mixture.
Spray both sides of coated tilapia with olive oil.
Bake on a rack on a cookie sheet in oven for 25 minutes at 400 degrees.
Serve with lemon wedges.

<u>Notes:</u>

Makes 4 servings

1.5 grams net carbs per serving .

Chicken Alfredo over Tofu Noodles

Ingredients:

4 boneless skinless chicken breasts
3 packages of Shirataki Tofu Noodles
Sauce:
- ½ cup of butter
- ½ cup of cream
- ¾ cup of parmesan or Romano
- ¼ cup gorgonzola
- ¼ cup white wine
- salt and pepper to taste

Directions:

Boil chicken in large pot for 25 minutes. Drain, cool, and, then with a fork and knife, pull apart into strips.

Wash tofu noodles in a strainer. Then, cook in medium sauce pan, uncovered over high heat.

In a separate sauce pan, melt butter over low to medium heat, add cream and cheese. Once cheese is melted, stir in the remaining sauce ingredients. Mix well. Then, add in chicken strips.

Serve chicken Alfredo sauce over tofu noodles.

Notes:

Makes 6 servings

3 grams net carbs per serving

Emily's Quick Chicken Pizzaiola

Ingredients:

1 1/4lb boneless skinless chicken breast -- cooked & shredded

Whole grain, light bread (<6 g carb per slice) or Dreamfields Penne

Sauce:

- 3 tbsp olive oil
- 1 cup yellow onion – finely chopped
- 2 garlic cloves – minced
- 1 ½ cups tomato sauce
- ½ cup dry red wine
- ½ tsp salt
- 1 ½ teaspoons dried oregano
- ½ tsp dried basil
- ½ tsp Italian seasoning
- 1/8 tsp crushed red pepper flakes

Directions:

In large pot, boil chicken breasts for 20 minutes, drain chicken, let cool, and then shred.

In a separate large saucepan, sauté the onion and garlic in oil until soft, but not browned.

Add tomato sauce, wine, oregano, basil, Italian seasoning, salt, and red pepper flakes.

Lower heat and simmer mixture for 30 minutes.

Add shredded, cooked chicken to the tomato sauce, and simmer together for 1 hour (Cover mixture if it begins to become too thick.).

Serve with melted cheese on low carb bread or tofu noodles.

Notes:

Makes 6 servings

10 grams net carbs per serving

Oven-Baked Shrimp

<u>Ingredients:</u>

2 pounds of cooked and peeled frozen shrimp.
2 tbsp. olive oil
salt and pepper

<u>Directions:</u>

Rinse shrimp and pat dry.
Mix shrimp with olive oil to coat.
Sprinkle with salt and pepper.
Place shrimp on a rack on a foil-lined cookie sheet.
Bake in oven for 7 minutes at 400 degrees.

<u>Notes:</u>

Serves 4

Excellent as a main course or on salad.

Pan Seared Shrimp

Ingredients

32 jumbo raw shrimp (21 to 25 shrimp per pound),
peeled, cleaned, and dried
½ cup flour
2 tbsp. olive oil
salt
pepper
1 tbsp. chopped fresh parsley
2 tbsp. butter

Directions:

Dust shrimp lightly with flour.
Heat oil in large electric skillet at medium high heat.
Add shrimp.
Season with salt and pepper. Then, Cover.
After 3 minutes, turn.
Cook 3 minutes longer.
Add butter and parsley.
Cook for 2 more minutes.

Note:

Serves 4

11 grams net carbs per serving

Easy Creamy Macaroni and Cheese

<u>Ingredients:</u>

½ cup dry Dreamfields elbows or 1 packet of tofu noodles
1 packet of Kraft Macaroni N Cheese, cheese powder mix
2 tbsp cream cheese
1 pre-cooked, grilled chicken breast (optional)

<u>Directions:</u>

Boil noodles in small sauce pan and drain.
Add cheese powder and cream cheese. Mix well.
Heat chicken, dice into small squares. Fold into mac n cheese.

<u>Notes:</u>

Makes 2 mini meal servings

Each serving contains approx. 4 g net carbs with Dreamfields elbows or 2 g net carbs with tofu noodles.

Supreme Personal Pizza

Ingredients:

½ of a light whole wheat English muffin
1 ounce tomato sauce
¼ cup of shredded Italian blend cheeses
Pepperoni, sausage, chicken or beef topping
Broccoli, mushrooms, zucchini, peppers or your choice of vegetable topping

Directions:

Cover English muffin with sauce, cheese, meat and vegetable toppings
Place on baking sheet in oven at 375 degrees until cheese is melted and browned.

Notes:

Makes 1 serving.

10 grams net carbs per serving

Sauces

Cheese Sauce

Ingredients:

3 tbsps. melted butter
2 cups shredded sharp cheddar cheese
1 cup sour cream
¼ tsp. salt
¼ tsp black pepper
¼ tsp. cayenne pepper (red pepper)
1 tsp. dried parsley

Directions:

Heat all ingredients in a pan until melted.

Note:

Makes 8 servings

2 grams net carbs per serving

Cheese Sauce (Alternate)

Ingredients:

2 tbsp. butter
2 tbsp. flour
¼ tsp. salt
dash of white pepper
1 cup half and half
1 cup shredded sharp cheddar cheese

Directions:

Melt butter over medium heat.
Stir in flour, salt, and a dash of pepper.
Wisk in 1 cup of half and half.
Stir in cheddar cheese.

Serve over steamed vegetables or chicken.

Note:
Makes six ¼-cup servings.

4 grams net carbs per serving

Low-Carb BBQ Sauce

Ingredients:

¾ cup of chopped onion
2 tbsp. olive oil
½ tsp. garlic salt
¼ tsp. salt
¼ tsp. pepper
1 ½ cups of diet cola (sweetened with Splenda—not aspartame)
1 6-oz. can of tomato paste
1 tbsp. white vinegar
3 packets of Truvia
3 tbsp. mustard
1 tbsp. soy sauce
a pinch of cloves
3 dashes of hot sauce

Directions:

In sauce pan, sauté onions in olive oil.
Add remaining ingredients and stir.
Cover and Simmer for 30 minutes on low heat, stirring occasionally.

Notes:

Makes six ¼-cup servings

3 grams net carbs per serving

Use on ribs or chicken.

Sauce can be made in advance and stored in refrigerator for up to a week.

Do not use diet cola with aspartame (Nutra Sweet or Equal). It can be toxic if heated.

Thickening Gravies, Sauces, and Soups with Alternatives to Flour

Use Xanthan Gum:

- Put Xanthan Gum in a pepper shaker.
- Shake it lightly into the liquid being thickened.
- As you shake in the Xanthan Gum, whisk vigorously.
- Repeat shakes and stirring, until it starts to thicken.
- It will get even thicker after you stop adding the powder.

Use Guar Gum:

- Mix 2 tsp. guar gum with ½ cup of cold water.
- Whisk it into 1 quart of simmering gravy, sauce, or soup.

Each thickening agent has zero net carbs.

Breakfast

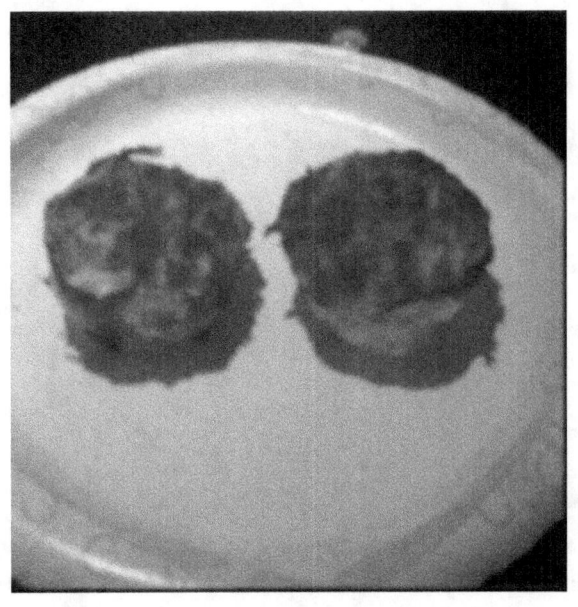

Yo'tmeal

Ingredients:

¼ cup all natural plain yogurt or Greek 1 packet Truvia (if using unsweetened protein powder)

OR

1 container of Dannon Carb Control vanilla yogurt (3 g carbs)

PLUS...

¼ cup ground Anutra or ground flax

1 serving unsweetened plain whey protein powder (Thin uses Biochem Greens and Whey – vanilla flavored.)

1 tbsp. olive oil

Directions:

Mix all ingredients in a cereal bowl.

Note:

1 bowl of yo'tmeal:

7 grams net carbs per serving if using regular plain yogurt

4 grams net carbs per serving if using Dannon Carb Control or Greek yogurt

<u>Option:</u>

Add 1 tsp. of cinnamon

Ham and Egg Cups

Ingredients:

2 thin slices of ham or Canadian bacon
2 eggs
salt and pepper
1 tbsp. shredded cheddar cheese
olive oil spray

Directions:

Spray 2 sections of muffin tin with olive oil.
Press a slice of ham or Canadian bacon into each section, forming a cup.
Put one raw egg into each cup.
Top each egg with salt, pepper, and a little cheese.
Bake at 400 degrees for 15 minutes.
Remove from oven and wait 5 minutes.
Loosen sides with a butter knife and serve.

Notes:

1 serving

This recipe is great for holiday brunches.

Make extras to refrigerate or freeze for future quick lunches.

Perfect Protein Shake

<u>Ingredients:</u>

4 ice cubes
1 scoop protein powder (1)
1 scoop Anutra
½ cup frozen berries (6)
½ cup unsweetened almond milk (1)
Stevia to taste

<u>Directions:</u>

Add all ingredients into blender. Blend until desired consistency.

<u>Notes:</u>

Makes 1 serving

8 grams net carbs per serving

Raspberry Velvet Smoothie

Ingredients:

4 ice cubes
1 scoop protein powder
1 cup fresh raspberries
½ cup unsweetened almond milk
1 tbsp. of unsweetened cocoa powder
3-4 packets of sweetener (Stevia, Truvia, or Splenda)

Directions:

Add all ingredients into blender. Blend until desired consistency.

Notes:

Makes 1 serving

12 grams net carbs per serving

Detox Smoothie

<u>Ingredients:</u>

4 ice cubes
1 scoop protein powder (1 g carbs)
1 scoop Anutra
½ cup unsweetened soy milk or almond milk (2 g carbs)
1to 2 oz. herbal aloe vera or acai berry juice (2 g carbs)
Stevia to taste

<u>Directions:</u>

Add all ingredients into blender. Blend until desired consistency.

<u>Notes:</u>

Makes 1 serving

5 grams net carbs per serving

Low-Carb French Toast

Ingredients:

2 slices light bread (6 net carbs or less per slice)

Batter:
- 2 eggs
- 1 oz. half n half
- 1 tsp. cinnamon
- 1 packet of Splenda or Truvia
- Salt and pepper to taste

Directions:

Mix all batter ingredients together in bowl.
Dip bread in batter mix, making sure both sides are fully coated.
Cook on skillet over medium heat, until golden brown.
Top with butter and or sugar free syrup.

Notes:

Makes 1 serving

14 grams net carbs per serving

Cinnamon Toast

<u>Ingredients:</u>

1 slice whole wheat, light bread (up to 9 g net carbs)
1 tbsp. butter
liberal amount of cinnamon
1 packet of Truvia

<u>Directions:</u>

Toast bread until crispy.
Melt butter on toast and spread.
Sprinkle Truvia over toast (Truvia gives a brown-sugar like texture.).
Top with a generous amount of cinnamon.

<u>Notes:</u>

Makes 1 serving

12 grams net carbs per serving

Sausage Egg and Cheese Breakfast Sandwich

<u>Ingredients:</u>

1 whole wheat English muffin
1 egg
1 all natural, nitrate-free sausage paddy
1 slice of cheddar cheese

<u>Directions:</u>

Toast English muffin in toaster
Cook egg (over hard) and sausage on skillet
Place on toasted English muffin
Add cheese

<u>Notes:</u>

Makes 2 servings.

8 grams net carbs per serving

Snacks

Warm Home-Made Cheese Crackers

Ingredients:

slices of cheddar cheese

Directions:

Arrange cheese slices on a non-stick frying pan or griddle.
Turn on the heat to medium-high.
When bottom of cheese is solid and golden brown, turn cheese with a spatula.
Continue to heat until the cheese turns into a solid cracker.
Place hot cheese crackers on paper towels.

Mini Pizza Snacks

Ingredients:

3 The Kitchen Table Bakers Hand Made Gourmet
Wafer Crisps*
1 oz. provolone cheese
3 pepperoni slices

Directions:

Put 3 crisps on a microwavable safe plate.
Top each crisp with cheese and a slice of pepperoni.
Microwave for 25 seconds.

Notes:

Makes 1 serving

The 3 wafer crisps (collectively) contain the following:

1 gram net carb per serving

*These cheese wafers are sold at Wegman's Grocery
Store. See website below to order online or to read
about them being featured on Rachel Ray's show.

http://www.kitchentablebakers.com/

Chocolate Coconut Candy

Ingredients:

1 jar of almond butter (12 oz.)
1 bar Ghiradelli 100 % cacao (unsweetened)
1 cup of hazelnut flour
1 cup of unsweetened shredded coconut
30 packets Truvia

Directions:

Microwave almond butter and cacao for 90 seconds.
Add flour, coconut, and Truvia.
Mix.
Spoon into 40 mini muffin cups.
Freeze.

Notes:

Makes about 40 cookies.

4.5 grams net carbs per serving

Chocolate Candy

<u>Ingredients:</u>

10 oz. bag Ghiradelli 100 % Cacao or other unsweetened chocolate chips for baking
(or 1 Ghiradelli 100 % Cacao bar)
12 oz. jar creamy almond butter
30 packets of Truvia

<u>Directions:</u>

In a bowl, melt chocolate and almond butter in
microwave for 90 seconds.
Add Truvia and stir.
Pour mixture into a 8 X 8 non-stick square pan or 42
mini muffin cups.
Freeze.

<u>Note:</u>

The chocolate can be eaten frozen or thawed.

Serving size: 1 piece

4 grams net carbs per serving

Cannoli Snack Mix

<u>Ingredients:</u>

½ cup part-skim ricotta cheese
¼ scoop of protein powder
2 packets of Splenda, Truvia or liquid Stevia
Dash of cinnamon or unsweetened cocoa powder
(optional)

<u>Directions:</u>

Place ricotta in small but deep bowl, add protein powder and sweetener. Mix well and top with cinnamon or cocoa powder.

<u>Notes:</u>

Makes 1 serving

6 grams net carbs per serving

12 grams net carbs per serving with Truvia)

Chocolate Mousse

Ingredients:

¼ cup yogurt (3 g carbs)
1 tbsp peanut butter (2 g carbs)
2 tbsp unsweetened cocoa powder (4 g carbs)
1 packet of Stevia and 1 packet of Truvia (3 g carbs)

Directions:

Place cocoa powder and peanut butter in small bowl. Then, heat in microwave for 30 seconds.

Add yogurt and sweetener, then blend thoroughly.

Notes:

Makes 1 serving

12 grams net carbs per serving

Peanut Butter and Jelly Sandwich

Ingredients:

1 slice light bread (6 net carbs or less per slice)
1 tbsp peanut butter
1 tbsp sugar free jam

Directions:

Make as you would a normal peanut butter and jelly sandwich.

Notes:

Makes 1 serving

10 grams net carbs per serving

Stuffed Banana Peppers

Ingredients:

½ small white onion chopped
1 small tomato chopped
1 medium bell pepper chopped
2 cups grated mixed cheeses
1 jalapeno pepper chopped
¼ lb. bacon
1 doz. banana peppers, seeds removed

Directions:

Broil bacon until crispy.

Mix all ingredients together except for banana peppers.

Wash and remove stem and seeds from banana peppers. Then, stuff with mixed ingredients.

Cover ends with tinfoil to prevent the mixture from spilling out when melted.

Bake in pan for 30-40 minutes at 375 degrees.

Notes:

Makes 12 servings

Contains approx. 0 net carbs*

*excluding veggies

Beverages

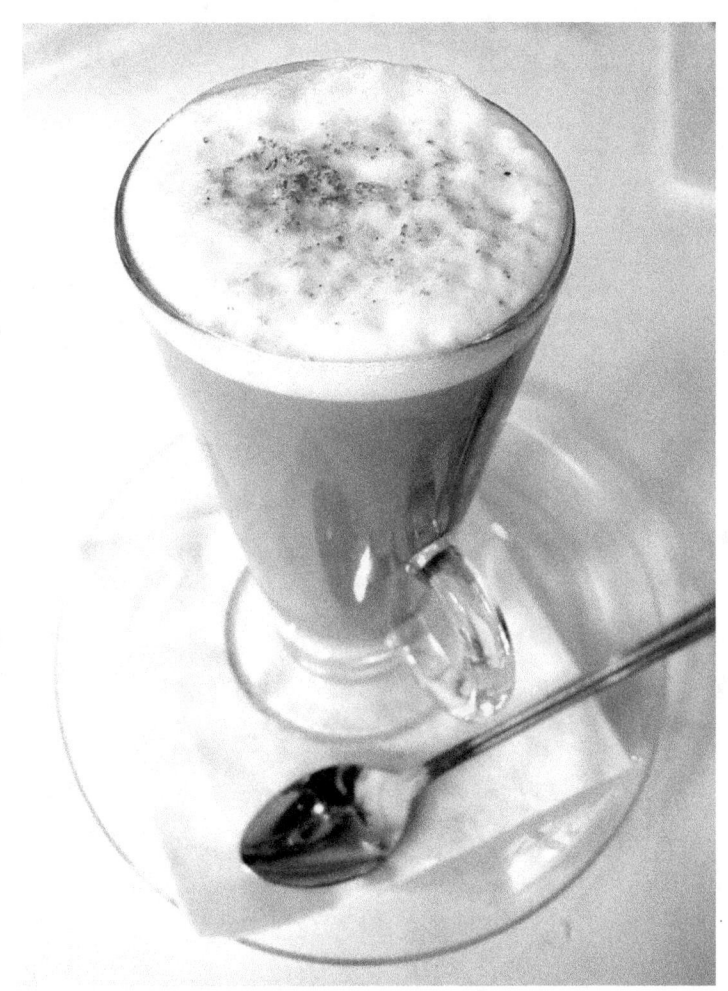

Café Mocha

Ingredients:

1 packet sugar free / diet hot cocoa mix (3 g of carbs)
½ cup coffee
¼ cup half n half
whipped cream (optional)

Directions:

Pour packet of hot cocoa mix into coffee mug, add coffee and stir. In a separate mug heat half n half in microwave for 30 seconds then pour and stir into the coffee/cocoa blend. Top with whipped cream and you've got yourself a coffee house classic.

Notes:

Makes 1 serving

5 grams net carbs per serving

Chai Tea

<u>Ingredients:</u>

1 black or green tea bag
¼ cup half n half
5 drops liquid Stevia
1 cinnamon stick

<u>Directions:</u>

Pour boiling water over tea bag, add half n half. Stir in Stevia. Then, stir with cinnamon stick.

<u>Notes:</u>

Makes one serving

2 grams net carbs per serving

Skinny Chocolate Milk Shake

<u>Ingredients:</u>

4 ice cubes
1 scoop protein powder
½ cup unsweetened almond milk
1 tbsp. of unsweetened cocoa powder
3-4 packets of sweetener (Stevia, Truvia, or Splenda)
½ cup plain yogurt (optional for extra thick and creamy)

<u>Directions:</u>

Add all ingredients into blender. Blend until desired consistency.

<u>Notes:</u>

Makes 1 serving

12 grams net carbs per serving with yogurt

6 grams net carbs per serving without yogurt

www.ingramcontent.com/pod-product-compliance
Lightning Source LLC
Chambersburg PA
CBHW060245290526
45789CB00001B/200